CALM
in the Midst of **CHAOS**

Dr. Calm's Prescription
for Stress-Free Living

CALM

in the Midst of **CHAOS**

KIRAN DINTYALA, MD, MPH, ABIHM

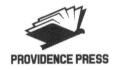

PROVIDENCE PRESS

TABLE OF CONTENTS

Part I: The Science of Inner Happiness

Part II: Stress—The Health Epidemic of the 21st Century

Part III: Understanding Stress and Debunking the Myths

Part IV: Discover the Forces that Shape Your Destiny

Part V: Exploring The P-E-T System: Your Ultimate Solution for Stress

Part VI: Moving Beyond Your Limitations

Part VII: Mastering the Big Three of Your Life: Time, Money, and Relationships

FOREWORD

D r. Kiran Dintyala has mastered the art of staying calm in the midst of chaos. Faced with great stresses that usually make a person anxious and depressed, he found a way to calm these emotions and discovered the secrets of inner happiness. Over time, Dr. Dintyala has developed a deep understanding of stress and its impact on the human mind and body, and a foolproof system for staying calm.

Calm in the Midst of Chaos shows the reader that happiness is our true inner nature. There is an epidemic of stress today with divisive politics, climate change, superstorms causing great damage, and growing nonsensical violence. General anxiety is rampant. A calm person is likely to survive and succeed during these stressful times more than anyone else. This book shows you how.

I have more than 40 years practicing and teaching Family Medicine with a deep understanding of behavioral science. I learned much from reading and reflecting on this book. It is like having a cognitive behavioral therapist, a physician, and a wellness coach in your home as you read. *Calm in the Midst of Chaos* will give you insights into stress, being calm, and happiness that are likely to result in new knowledge and understanding. There are many myths and common false understandings of stress today that Dr. Dintyala dispels with empathy and compassion.

The P-E-T system and other tools in the book are the best guides I know for stress-free living and will serve you for the rest of your life. Leonardo da Vinci and Steve Jobs are famous for saying that simplicity is the ultimate sophistication. Simple rules are regarded as the best method for dealing with complexity in life. In *Calm in the Midst of Chaos,* you will find that simplicity. It may be the most important book you will read in many years. Enjoy it and learn from it.

Joseph E. Scherger, MD, MPH
Vice President, Primary Care and Academic Affairs
Eisenhower Medical Center, Rancho Mirage, CA

ACKNOWLEDGMENTS

First and foremost, I acknowledge the fact that I wouldn't have been able to write a single word of inspiration without the intuitive guidance provided by God and the teachings of my guru Sri Paramahansa Yogananda. Their constant presence is the guiding force of my life and an eternal source of inspiration, strength, and courage to pursue all my endeavors.

I am deeply indebted to my parents and my sister for their steadfast love and support, without which I would not have developed into the person and professional I am today. I come from a middle-class family. My parents had daily financial struggles that lasted for years and sacrificed enormously to ensure I received a proper education.

My wife, Mariana, who believes in my knowledge and abilities, encouraged and supported me in writing this book in the first place. She is my strongest advocate and staunchest critic. Without her love, friendship, and companionship, it would not have been possible for this book to ever see the light of day.

Our daughter, Mayura, who gives meaning to my life, inspires me every day to progress and prosper in life. In her beautiful ways, she reminds me to live life to the fullest every moment.

Professor Judith Sedgeman deserves the most appreciation as the person who influenced me to pursue the path to stress freedom that I have undertaken. Undoubtedly, she is one of the most inspiring teachers I have ever encountered. She is an embodiment of the simplicity and wisdom of the Three Principles living. If not for meeting her early in my career, I would have taken a different path in life. My association with her initiated my exploration of the field of innate health and resiliency. I am deeply grateful for her guidance and help.

My thanks also to Dr. William Pettit for the many insights I have gained through his teachings of the Three Principles.

My dearest friend Nageswara Rao Karri has been a tremendous moral and intellectual support for me throughout the process of writing this book over a span of four years. His unwavering commitment to be my greatest supporter in this endeavor is invaluable and unmatched.

I am thankful to the editors and reviewers of this book who helped me journey through the writing of this book, my first one, and provided their endless support. Some of the people who helped me in this process are Dr. Sharon Diamen, Dr. Murthy Andavolu, Madalyn Stone, Brigitte Robindor'e, Deb Englander, and Heidi Grauel.

Last, but not least, a special thanks goes to Martha Bullen for her phenomenal guidance and for holding my hand at each step of the complex process of book publishing and leading me to successfully finish this book.

PREFACE

tress, stress, stress! We live in a world teeming with stress. It seems as ubiquitous as life itself. Millions of people across the globe experience deep distress every day. Stress has become an inevitable, toxic byproduct of fast-paced, modern living. The world itself has become a stress bomb ready to explode at any minute. Sexual abuse, alcoholism, terrorism, drug trafficking, gun violence, suicide bombings, and many other deeply rooted problems of our society are extreme manifestations of the profoundly dysfunctional state of mind, called *stress*. Our families, schools, workplaces, organizations, health care industry, political systems, and humankind as a whole are struggling helplessly to escape the deadly grip of stress. Even our very planet, Mother Earth, is experiencing unprecedented damage from human stress, seen in climate change, deforestation, chemical warfare, loss of biodiversity, severe water and air pollution, and overpopulation.

No matter how determined we are to lead a life of peace and joy, life's challenges constantly try to knock us off balance and steal our peace of mind. Often, we get entangled in a mix of negative emotions like worry, anxiety, and anger, or other forms of stress. Time and again, we find ourselves caught in ferocious stress storms that stir up chaos. Our very thoughts, actions, emotions, relationships, finances, and literally all aspects of our lives experience frequent turmoil. Billions of people around the world feel stuck in this vicious cycle of stress and wonder, "How can we put back our lives in balance? What should we do?

Frequently, during my seminars, people ask me how they can face the challenges of life with grace. They want to know how to lead a fulfilled life of peace and joy and how to maintain even-mindedness in the face of uncertainty. They wonder how we can exit this stress cycle and put our lives back in balance. Is it even possible? The simple answer is yes. The good news is that there are Universal Principles that help us understand our true selves, reclaim the lost joy and peace in our lives, and tap into our unlimited potential. And there are exercises and techniques that help us find calmness, dissolve stress, and stand victorious in life. I am not talking about merely coping with stress. There are many books for that. I am talking about *preventing*—and possibly eliminating—most stress from your life.

In this book, I present a powerful system to overcome stress, which I have named *The P-E-T System for Stress-Free Living*. This system is drawn from five major sources. First, in handling a variety of stressful situations in my personal life; second, from my professional life as a physician, with more than fifteen years of experience interacting with patients and observing the impact of stress on health and disease; third, from my exposure to the philosophy of *the Three Principles* as defined by Sydney Banks[1];

---

1 It's important to note that this book is written out of the inspiration drawn from the Three Principles as originally taught by the late Mr. Sydney Banks. This book reflects my own understanding of the Three Principles based on my own experiences and my perceptions of the effect of stress on human

fourth, from my study of the subject of innate health and resiliency while earning my master's degree in public health; fifth, and perhaps most significantly, from my deep study of the principles and science of yoga as taught by the Great Master Paramahansa Yogananda. By distilling the essence from all these sources and combining them with my life experiences, I was able to develop a system that has been put to the test and repeatedly proven to work. At the time of printing, preliminary test results of a six-month research program I have implemented, called *The Stress Mastery Program*, show that those who practice the P-E-T System have seen a significant reduction in their stress levels.

Why I Wrote This Book

Billions around the world find their endless efforts to attain peace, joy, and balance in life fruitless. It is because they were never taught the science and art of stress mastery at home, school, college, or work. Few people receive formal stress education in their life. If they did receive any lessons on stress reduction, they were taught superficial techniques that didn't address the root cause of stress in their lives.

Having experienced extremes of stress in my own life and learning the lessons of life the hard way, I hope to share my experiences and insights to help people experience less stress and more joy in their lives. Many times, what I call "the stress tiger" (see the Introduction) tried to eat me alive, but each time I emerged victorious. Soon, I realized that if I could learn the art of *taming the tiger* of stress, I no longer had to fear it. Over the years, I have put together all of my experiences and understanding of surviving

---

life. But, ultimately, the truth is that the Three Principles of Mind, Thought, and Consciousness are Universal, and they appear to vary or differ only to the degree of our own understanding. The greater your understanding of these Principles, the more you will see them as the foundational elements of all true teachings that bestow lasting happiness and peace of mind.

stress and living a peaceful and joyful life into a simple system that anyone can learn and follow.

Every day I see my patients, colleagues, friends, and family members stressed. I think to myself, *if they only knew the Principles and practices of P-E-T System, they could instantly be relieved of stress and find peace and joy!* In my desire to help them, I started sharing this knowledge. My work spread by word-of-mouth. Soon, I began offering workshops and was inspired to increase their frequency when I saw how much people were benefiting from them. Often, someone in the audience stood up right in the middle of my presentation and shared how it felt to be stress-free for the first time in many years, leaving behind worries and fears, ready to move forward in life. I decided to compile the principles and practices I teach in this book so that I could reach a broader audience.

As a physician and a public health professional, I would like to contribute to the betterment of the health of our society. In my practice, countless patients have expressed concerns about the devastating levels of stress in their lives. I could clearly see the impact of stress on our nation's health. Yet, our current health system offers no stress solutions that are readily available and easily accessible for the general population.

Fighting stress is at least as important, if not more important, as fighting cancer, heart disease, or other debilitating illnesses. In fact, my experience and observations have taught me that stress is at the root of almost all disease, and that its reduction and elimination are of the utmost priority for the well-being of humanity and, indeed, of all life on earth. There is a tremendous and pressing need to create stress solution tools and services for the benefit of the public at large. I decided to create them. And this book is one of them, along with audio, video, and live and online programs.

To the Reader

As you read through the book, first try to understand the material being discussed. Let the understanding sink deeply within you. Clarify your understanding by rereading and reviewing the material in the book. Ask one of your friends or relatives to pair up with you to learn, apply, and discuss the P-E-T System. That's the best way to maximize your learning from this book.

If you have questions, email us at *info@StressFreeRevolution. com* and we can help you.

As you discuss these teachings with others, questions will arise. Go back to the book and review the material. It will help you refine your learning and deepen your understanding. With practice, you will see the positive results of what you have learned, and you will want to share this exciting discovery with others. They will pose questions and you will try to find answers again. You will learn even more, gaining a new level of understanding. This upward spiral of learning, understanding, and teaching will continue. Soon, stress will exit your life though the back door, ever hesitant to return as long as you practice the P-E-T System steadfastly and anchor yourself strongly in calmness.

There are many positive results you will experience from practicing the material discussed in this book, and some of the key benefits include:

1. Turning off the stress alarm and developing stress resistance
2. Finding calm in the midst of chaos
3. Performing well, even under pressure, and increasing productivity
4. Resolving conflicts and building better relationships
5. Finding more time to do what matters most to you
6. Experiencing peace, joy, and balance in life
7. Improving health and sleep

Good books can elevate your life. During the times when you are unable to share your problems with friends and family or when they cannot provide you the answers you need, you can turn to books for help. Many times, in my own life, I found great advice and solace from reading good books. You can, too, if you follow the powerful principles and practices revealed in this book. After reading it, you will be able to access and utilize the power of *The P-E-T System for Stress-Free Living*. You don't have to take my word for it. Experiment for yourself. Give it a try; be patient, and you will be amazed by the tremendous positive impact it will have on your life. It will help you reclaim your equanimity and inner peace. You will find *calm in the midst of chaos*, regardless of the challenges you face. This system works in real time, in real life. Learn it, use it, and teach it. Not only will you transform your life, you will also profoundly affect those around you. You will become part of the growing movement I call *The Stress-Free Revolution*. Let's begin your journey.

The Tale of a Deadly Tiger and a Calm Elephant

By Kiran

*The backdrop of this fable is
a jungle full of wild animals.*

Once there was a ferocious tiger that was a terror to all the animals in the forest. The tiger would prowl every day and hunt for a meal to satisfy his hunger, and then he would lie down, resting until his hunger pains woke him, ready to hunt again.

One day, the tiger decided to kill a big elephant so that he could relish the meat for several days and save himself from hunting every day.

The hungry tiger waited for the elephant at the lake at the center of the forest and lunged at it, trying to go for a kill. However, the tiger was no match for the elephant's might and got badly trampled. Watching this scene, the rest of the animals laughed at the tiger's stupidity. The tiger fled, defeated but determined to come back with a better plan to attack the elephant.

The tiger ventured out into the far end of the forest to see if there were other tigers that could help him. Finally, at the edge of the forest, he saw two more tigers and convinced them of his plan to kill the elephant. But they also knew that, even for three tigers, an elephant could be a formidable opponent. To aid them in their conquest, the three tigers decided to bribe a monkey with a handful of bananas to distract the elephant while they attacked.

The owl of wisdom, perched on the branch of the tree under which this conversation took place, immediately reached out to her friend the elephant that night and informed him of the tigers' plot. They brainstormed, and the owl advised the elephant that his best bet to win the fight was to be in the lake in the middle of the forest.

But the elephant raised a concern: "Tigers can swim."

The owl replied, "Yes, they can, but they are not as good hunters when they swim. They are more dangerous when they are on the land than in water."

The elephant liked that idea and woke up early the next morning and hurriedly walked toward the lake. Not aware of the elephant's knowledge of the tigers' plot, the three tigers followed the elephant to the lake, thinking that the elephant was just thirsty and going to the lake to drink water. The elephant pretended he was not aware of the tigers' presence and feigned to drink water. The three tigers approached the elephant quietly to ambush him.

Remember, the monkey's job was to distract the elephant by getting on top of his head while the tigers attacked. However, the elephant, having known the plot, anticipated the monkey's tactic and cleverly used his trunk to subjugate the monkey right away, even before the tigers attacked him.

The three tigers were now a little wary to attack the powerful elephant, knowing that the distracter monkey had already been quickly dispatched. Nevertheless, they decided to try their luck. As they lunged forward, the elephant, using his powerful trunk, pumped a jet of water at the first tiger while using his heavy foot to stomp on the second. The third tiger attacked the elephant from behind, but the elephant swirled swiftly around and used its long, sharp tusks to injure the third. The first tiger, recovering from being blown away by the tremendous force of the water jet from the elephant's trunk, did not dare to come close to the elephant, watching the fate of the other two tigers.

Startled by the abrupt counterattack by the elephant, the three injured tigers fled far away from the lake, learning the lesson of their lives to never dare to attack an elephant! The elephant, unscathed by the fight, gracefully walked toward his dear friend the owl, perched on the branch of the nearby tree, to thank her for her words of wisdom that saved his life. They both laughed out loud and danced around happily, celebrating their victory.

Moral of the story:

In today's world, in the jungle of life, there are many ferocious tigers of stress waiting to attack our elephant of health. The monkeys of restless thoughts try to distract us incessantly, thus making us vulnerable. But the owl of wisdom that perches over the tree of calmness warns us of the dangers in the jungle of life. Using the mighty trunk of willpower, we have to subdue the monkey of restlessness.

With a calm mind, you can face the challenges of life with grace. A mind that is tranquil like a lake will safeguard you from tigers of stress. Watching the silent power of a calm mind, the tigers of stress will not dare to attack you anymore. But as soon as the monkey of restlessness succeeds in distracting us, the tigers of stress will rally back to bring down our elephant of health. *Calm the restless monkey mind and stand victorious against the tigers of stress!*

Great teachers say stress is an illusion, and it all originates from our insecure thoughts. I acknowledge the deep truth in that statement, but stress is not an illusion for countless people across this world who are not able to identify its true origin and who are incessantly struggling to find solace in their lives. For people who realize this deep truth—that stress stems from our insecure thinking—stress is a laughing matter and just an illusion; but for people who have not realized that truth, stress is a monster that exists outside their mind.

I hope this book takes you through a journey *from the belief that stress is a monster outside of you to the realization of this deep truth: stress is nothing but trivial thoughts of insecurity projected by your own mind, powerful enough to give the illusion that stress approaches you from the outside.*

PART I

The Science of Inner Happiness

Part I Objectives

- Discover your true nature, which is peace, joy, and contentment.
- Dispel doubts about your ability to overcome stress and find happiness in your life.
- Ignite your innate ability to recover from challenges and reestablish peace in your life.

CHAPTER 1

Peace of Mind Is Your True Nature

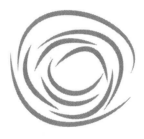

Like the eye of a hurricane, there is a sacred place of peace deep within you, untouched by the chaos around.

The King, the Sage, and the Science of Inner Happiness

Once there lived a noble king who wanted to lift everyone in his kingdom out of poverty and relieve their financial struggles so that they may live happily ever after. He had more than enough gold in his treasury to make every person in the kingdom wealthy for their entire lives. Six months later, he ventured out in disguise as a traveler to various corners of his kingdom to inquire about the happiness of his people. To his surprise, he discovered that most people in his kingdom were still deeply unhappy. Utterly confused by this phenomenon, the king continued his journey to the far ends of the kingdom, searching for answers. He met many intelligent people and scholars on his way, but none could answer his questions to satisfaction.

Finally, he came across a sage sitting under a tree in his hermitage. The king in disguise posed the same question to the sage. The sage replied, "Dear sir, you seem to be tired. Why don't you rest here as my guest for a few days? You can eat all you want and are free to spend time in my garden and roam in the nearby forest. My assistants will serve you, and all your material needs will be provided for here. I need to go to the nearby town on important work. Once I return, I will answer your question." The king, in need of rest, accepted the offer. Two weeks passed by and no sign of the sage still. Another week passed by, and still, the king saw no sign of the sage. A month passed by, and the impatient king saw no sign of the sage returning.

The king, extremely angry and upset, decided to leave the hermitage and summoned his soldiers to punish the sage for his disrespect toward him. Just when the king was about to step out of the hermitage, the sage returned. He saw that the king was wretched, more so than when he first came to the hermitage. The sage broke out in laughter, and the king, utterly perplexed by this strange behavior, asked him why he was laughing uncontrollably. The sage replied, "Dear sir, the answer to your question lies in the situation you are facing. I have provided you with everything you need at the hermitage, and you are still unhappy. Why is that? Isn't this situation like the one our king is facing?

"Our king thought that providing for material needs alone would keep people happy forever. The truth is that unless people learn the science of crafting inner happiness, they will only grow more and more impatient in their lives, asking for more and more material needs. The thirst for material desires can never be quenched, even with all the riches of the world, let alone the wealth in the kingdom. Like the wild tigers roaming in the jungle and causing distress to all the beings that come across their path, mental maladies like anger, greed, hate, and worry roam in the minds of people, causing them distress. These psychological stress tigers are far more dangerous and need to be knocked unconscious to prevent them from creating havoc in your mind before you can enjoy true happiness. This inner mastery of mind is the only true path to lasting happiness in life."

Listening to the sage's answer and experiencing the truth in his message, the king's face softened, with a gentle smile appearing on his countenance. He thanked the sage for his wise counsel and returned to his kingdom. He sent out an invitation to the sage to be his advisor and spread this message to liberate the people of his kingdom from the grip of psychological stress tigers.

This book teaches the science of inner happiness, and this chapter introduces you to innate health, which is the foundation for our inner happiness.

Innate Health

Peace of mind is your true nature. We all are born that way. No exceptions! Innate health is your natural state of mental well-being, where your happiness is unconditional and your peace of mind is boundless (see Figure 1.1). Within you, there is a strong undercurrent of peace, joy, and contentment, all regardless of your circumstances. That's your default setting. That's your true nature. It is not a characteristic inherited by a few people in the world. It's not limited to people who are physically strong. It is not related to how much money you have nor your aesthetics. It does not depend on any external conditions. It's a universal gift we are bestowed at birth. It has been, and will continue to be there, waiting to be realized. Deep inside, it remains untainted, despite all the stresses of life. It is this innate health that makes it possible for you to remain unruffled even during the greatest challenges of life.

> Peace of mind is your true nature. We all are born that way. No exceptions!

Your Happiness Is Conditioned as You Grow into Adulthood

Children are perfect examples of innate health. They are playful, joyful, and naturally adorable; when something bad happens, they cry for a few minutes and then come back to their normal selves quickly and continue to play. As we grow into adulthood, we condition our happiness to certain things, whether it is money, fame, a desired job, or something else, and think that we can't be happy without it. But we all know that we were happy when we were younger. It didn't matter our skin color, whether we had one toy or ten, or whether we were rich or poor. But soon that child gets trained by parents, family, friends, and the environment to be happy only under certain conditions. As we grow older, we add more of those conditions to achieve happiness in our lives. The more conditions we have to satisfy to become happy, the harder it is for us to be happy.

Do Not Make "If" a Determinant of Your Happiness

There are many things that can potentially condition your happiness—your environment, society, culture, parents, family, friends, school, social media, and so on. You may easily slip into the trap of limiting your happiness to certain circumstances or

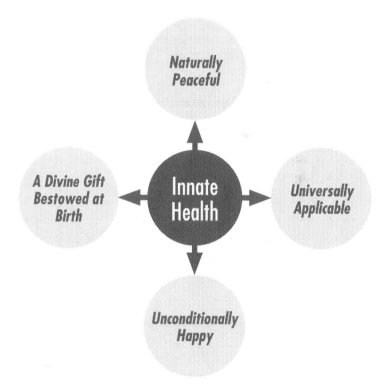

Figure 1.1. Innate Health — Key Characteristics

achievements; this is called conditional happiness. In conditional happiness, "if" becomes a major determinant of your happiness. You think, "I can be happy if I get a new bicycle" or "if I get a new job" or "if I live in Hawaii" or if something else! Some of these desires and goals are very realistic. And there is nothing wrong in setting goals and achieving them. In fact, you should set goals because in that process, you learn, grow, and tap into your unknown potentials. However, the problems arise when you forget that true happiness lies within and you identify your happiness with specific circumstances or conditions. That mistaken identity of happiness depletes the joy in your life, and soon stress finds the doorway into your existence!

The Seed of Unhappiness

This misidentification or misconnection of your happiness with external circumstances is the seed of unhappiness. Often, these seeds were sown in your mind by social and environmental conditioning while you were still a small child. These seeds of unhappiness, the ideas that you need something else to make you happy, hide beneath the fertile soil of your mind until the conditions are favorable for them to grow. With time, these seeds grow into a big tree of life with many branches of desires with myriad fruits of outcomes—a tree that you climb to grab those fruits. Soon, you realize that on the tree of life there are an infinite number of fruits with varied tastes and flavors that you feel compelled to taste. Then life becomes a fruit race, and you become a fruit ninja, trying to slice and taste one fruit of desire after another forever.

Do Not Become Too Engrossed in the Game of Life

In this process, you become so engrossed in the "game of life" that your happiness becomes completely entangled with your desires, goals, and outcomes. But when your efforts to accomplish these objectives are thwarted, you become unhappy, angry, upset, or distressed. Also, when you lose the material possessions you accumulated, you become anxious. You live at this level of stressful thinking, forgetting that once upon a time you were unconditionally happy without being affected by any of these worldly ambitions and were strongly anchored to the joy and peace within yourself—your natural state of mind. You forget that your innate health is perfectly preserved within, no matter what your external circumstances might look like. The following story demonstrates the limitless nature of desires and the risk associated with relentlessly chasing them.

The Mystic Tree of Desires

Once there was a mystic tree, heavy with different kinds of fruits on its branches. It had apples, pears, mangoes, oranges, berries, and every other fruit imaginable. A man and his teenage boy passed by, and the boy wanted to climb the tree and taste the fruits. The man warned the boy not to and said the tree is full of illusions. But the boy didn't heed the advice and climbed the tree when his father was not around. As he climbed the tree, he discovered that there were all kinds of fruits, just as he read in the book of mysteries.

He picked the nearest mango and found that it was the most delicious mango he had ever tasted. Then right next to it was a white apple and next to that was a red orange. He quickly devoured them and surprisingly noticed that instead of feeling full in the stomach, he felt hungrier than ever. Then he saw a variety of berries and a large watermelon on the branch next to him. He quickly swallowed a bunch of berries and opened the melon to quench his thirst and satisfy his hunger. And, once again, surprisingly, he found his appetite insatiable and his thirst unquenchable.

By this time, his father had come back from work, found his lad all the way up in the tree, and called him down. But the curious teen wanted to demystify the mysteries of the tree, and he climbed on. There he found a shiny black fruit, something he had never seen before, nestled far away from his reach. He carefully crawled closer to it and when he was just about to lay his hands on the fruit, out of nowhere a giant snake with three heads appeared and struck him hard on his neck. Crying out loud in pain, losing control, the boy—without tasting the black fruit—fell all the way down, almost losing his consciousness when his father came to his rescue and saved his life.

After the poison was taken out and the boy recuperated, his father lovingly asked, "Did you find what you want up there?" The boy answered, "No." "Do you think you are ever going find what you want on that tree of illusion?" The boy answered, "I don't know." The father explained, "You wouldn't. It's because on this mystical tree of illusion, every fruit you desire only increases your hunger. No matter how many fruits you taste, your desire for more will never be satisfied."

Moral of the Story

Life is like a tree of illusion. Material desires are like those imagined fruits. No matter how many material desires you pursue, none of them are going to make you completely happy. You will feel like you always need more of something. That goes on until the snake of failure bites you hard and makes you fall. But you don't have to wait until the snake of failure bites you. You could wake up from the delusion before a tragedy like that happens in your life. Pursue your inner happiness, and all else will be added unto you.

The fruits on the tree are an illusion; in the same way, the snake is also an illusion and so the pain caused by the snake bite. Once you come out of the illusion you will not be either overcome by the desire for the fruits nor by the fear of the snake. You will learn to remain neutral to all temptations, lures, and disappointments of life.

Wake Up to Reality and Reclaim Your Happiness

The good news is you can reclaim your happiness without conditions. You can resolve past hurt, you can forgive and forget mistakes done by others who harmed you, you can dissolve the fear of the future, and you can undo all the conditions in your life and anchor yourself in a state of peace, joy, and contentment. In fact, the happiness that is lost is your conditional happiness. It is clear that, deep inside, your unconditional happiness—your innate health—remains untouched and untainted.

Do Not Wait Until the Snake of Failure Strikes You

Sometimes, reclaiming your unconditional happiness occurs automatically when you experience deep suffering. You suddenly realize that your happiness lies within, untainted by the circumstances. But you don't have to wait to experience failure or suffering before you start learning this truth. Start your journey to find unconditional happiness, your innate health, right now. Yes, I mean right now! Understanding and practicing the P-E-T System for Stress-Free Living is the gateway to peace and joy! Once you practice it, you will realize that you never lost your inner peace and joy . . . you only thought you lost it!

DR. CALM'S PRESCRIPTION

1 ✓ Realize that your true nature is one of peace, joy, and contentment.

2 ✓ Innate health is your natural state where your happiness is unconditioned and your peace of mind boundless.

3 ✓ During times of adversity, your conditional happiness is lost but deep within, your unconditional happiness—your innate health—remains intact and untouched.

4 ✓ Innate health is not dependent on external conditions such as money, race, country, or age. It is a divine gift bestowed at birth and maintained throughout life.

5 ✓ All the ups and downs in life can be compared to the waves of the ocean at the surface. Deep underneath the waves, the ocean is vast and remains undisturbed, much in the same way that deep within, the "True You" is not affected by the superficial, tumultuous events of life.

6 ✓ Do not link your happiness to external conditions. This is the root cause of all misery. Enjoy everything in life without being engrossed in them.

7 ✓ At every dark corner of life there is a snake of failure waiting to strike. Awaken yourself now to the light of reality before the snake of failure strikes you. It's much harder to learn and reform yourself under the spell of failure when you are being tested by life than when conditions are happier and conducive to growth. Wake up now before it is too late!

CHAPTER 2

The Power of Human Resilience

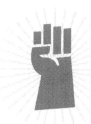

The indomitable nature of human resilience has been proven time and again through the ages. This power of resilience is yours to tap into, anytime you want.

Life Is a Series of Challenges

Sometimes, nothing seems to go in the right direction in life; as hard as you try, more challenges surface. As soon as you feel you solved one problem, another erupts from nowhere. During these times, you wonder, "Am I ever going to be peaceful? When will I get a respite from these endless trials?" Recently,

I experienced such a situation. During that time, the stress tiger relentlessly attacked me with one powerful blow after another, trying to unsettle and dismantle my life. Read on to discover how the power of resilience helped me overcome the challenges and restore my peace of mind.

A couple of years ago, I received a phone call from my uncle in India conveying the news that my father had experienced a life-threatening accident. I immediately flew to India. When I arrived, I found my dad fighting death after an accident that resulted in severe bleeding and multiple fractures. After two months of enormous struggle, his condition finally started to improve. With great relief, I booked a flight back to the United States. By that time, I had already been on a leave of absence from my job for more than two months. It was important that I return to the United States as soon as possible and resume my job right away.

In addition, my savings were running low, and I desperately needed to go back to work and make some money. That night, after paying a farewell visit to my family members, I departed for the airport. It was around midnight. I walked toward the airline kiosk, dragging three pieces of heavy luggage. The airline staff, after asking me a few questions, denied my departure that night. They said they couldn't let me fly because of a problem with my travel documents and visa. I was aghast at hearing that.

"What the hell? What's going on here? I never ran into this kind of problem before," I protested. My prolonged discussions with the airline personnel were not fruitful.

All night, I was running around to work things out,

but my efforts were in vain. Finally, mentally and physically exhausted, around 4 a.m., I decided to return home. I had to cancel my trip, and I was concerned whether my employer would allow me to extend my leave of absence. I came home and urgently applied for a new visa that morning. Usually, it takes four to five days to get a visa, but for some strange reason, my case was prolonged. I was informed that my case was sent for administrative processing and that it might take up to eight weeks before a final decision was made!

Negative thoughts enveloped me like a storm: "Usually, it only takes a few days to grant a visa. Why is this taking so long? What happens if my visa gets rejected? What happens if I'm not allowed back into the United States again? My seemingly prosperous career that I have built over many years will end abruptly."

While I was in the middle of dealing with this difficult issue, I received a message from one of my clients that they couldn't wait anymore for me to return to the United States and were withdrawing from a joint venture that was a golden opportunity for my career. A few other mishaps occurred successively, one after another around the same time, that didn't give me any breathing room to recover. All these challenges (there were six major challenges I was facing at that time, with many other minor problems also trying to wrest away my peace of mind) were occurring as if to test my resilience and my capability to remain calm in the midst of chaos. It's as if I had vanquished one stress tiger only to find that there is another leaping on me from behind, and then another and then another. I was being pushed to the limits.

At that time, I counseled myself, "It's all right! We can't control all the events in life. Life is a roller-coaster ride. There are times you will be at the peak of the ride and times you will be at the bottom. Just enjoy the ride. Do not let the momentary ups and downs in life destroy your confidence, strength, and faith. Just sit tight and let the situation pass. Allow your mind to be quiet. Allow the negative thoughts to pass and vanish. *If you allow yourself to be calm through these tough times, soon the downturn will pass, and the upturn will arrive.* Just enjoy the ride." With that self-counsel, my mind found the quiet it needed. I wrote down the list of things to be done, including which issues were under my control and which I did not have control over. Those things I couldn't control, I had to let go. Those things I could control, I worked on. The visa situation got resolved within a few days (instead of the four to eight weeks according to the original notice). Those few days were extra time to spend with family. My work situation turned out to be fine, too. In the end, everything was okay.

Once again, although life tested me very severely throughout those three extremely tough months, it also proved to me that with strong willpower and a calm mind, you can overcome the challenges. And it is possible because we are innately resilient as human beings.

The Power of Resilience

In life, we all go through difficult situations. As much as you try to remain at peace with yourself and the world around you, you are constantly pulled into rough situations that test your patience and character. It is as if someone is continuously trying to throw you off

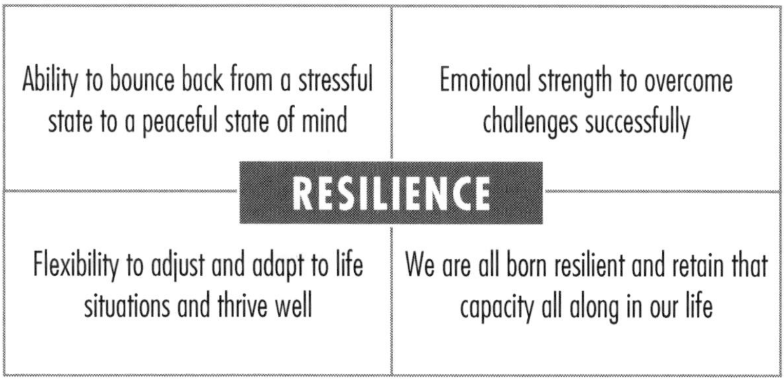

Ability to bounce back from a stressful state to a peaceful state of mind	Emotional strength to overcome challenges successfully
RESILIENCE	
Flexibility to adjust and adapt to life situations and thrive well	We are all born resilient and retain that capacity all along in our life

Figure 2.1. Resilience – Key Characteristics

balance. You often wonder, "Is there a way around it? Is there a way to handle these challenges gracefully and emerge victoriously?" Yes, there is a way! As a resilient being, you are inherently designed to win. *Even though you have no control over what life throws at you, you have control over your ability to respond.* You can choose your responses wisely. Your mind is strong, powerful, and flexible, giving you the ability to successfully overcome life's struggles. That's called *resilience*, and it gives us a fair degree of control over our lives(see Figure 2.1).

Resiliency is your capacity to recover and heal, to be flexible with life, and to recalibrate yourself and reclaim your lost joy, peace, and contentment in life.

> Even though you have no control over what life throws at you, you have control over your ability to respond. You can choose your responses wisely.

Resiliency is your capacity to revert from a stressful state of mind to a calm state of mind. It is your innate potential to rebalance and restore peace, regardless of your circumstances. *Being at peace and being joyful is your default setting. The very fact that this is your default state of mind makes it possible for you to recover from any kind of stress in life.* We all have the capability within us to be resilient, and we all can recover from even the worst situations of our lives.

Below is an example of a person who demonstrated extraordinary resilience despite trying circumstances and thus was able to access his innate health, peace of mind, and positive feelings.

I was hesitant to enter the room. I was not sure how to convey the horrible news to my patient. He was a pleasant, elderly man who had come into the hospital because he noticed blood in his urine. We ordered some tests and found a mass in his urinary bladder, which looked like bladder cancer. Even worse, further scans showed that the cancer might have spread to his bones, lungs, and other parts of his body. But we were not sure yet, so we ordered some biopsies from his bladder and lung.

The final test results confirmed our suspicion of cancer. But it was much worse than we initially suspected. He not only had bladder cancer but also lung cancer. And he had been in perfect health just a couple of weeks earlier. How devastating for anyone, going from perfect health to being diagnosed with multiple cancers within a matter of two weeks!

How do I break this terrible news? My medical students and I were all feeling badly for him and deeply sympathetic. I took a deep breath and went into his room. There he was, lying down on his bed, happy as always and reading a novel. I greeted him and sat in the chair next to him. We chatted a little bit about the book he was reading and how suspenseful it was.

Then, gathering all my courage and holding back my emotions, I whispered in a low voice, "I have bad news to share."

He looked at me with a smile and nodded his head that I could give the news. I told him that he had cancer in two separate organs and it had already spread to other areas in his body.

I paused for a moment and looked into his eyes. I was not sure whether it was because my eyes were tearful or the light in the room was dim and foggy, but everything looked hazy. Through that foggy vision, I could not believe what I saw. He was still smiling. I cleared my eyes and still saw that this great old man was still smiling. There was not even a hint of worry or unhappiness or anxiety in his demeanor.

He understood my struggle and said, "What can I do? If I get worried and get anxious, the cancer is not going to disappear. Then why worry about it? Let's fight it the best we can. If I am lucky, I will survive. If not, it's all right."

I was shocked by his complete and utter acceptance of the situation. How can a person be so calm, positive, and unruffled during such an inopportune time? That's the hallmark of a person who is very resilient. His innate mental health was perfectly intact despite his physical health being adversely affected by disease.*

---

* I report with great sadness that this gentleman, after a strong and heroic struggle fighting his cancer, did ultimately, with much grace, pass away after a few months. He maintained the same cheerful attitude until the last day of his life. I was proud to have him as my patient. People like him are the kind of people who give strength to us doctors. They serve as an inspiration to all of us. Every day, as doctors, we have to convey bad news to many patients. And, sometimes, just when we feel our emotional strength is fading, people like him energize and rejuvenate us with their tremendous positive energy. He is the best example of someone who has perfectly preserved innate health. Regardless of what's going on around and to him, he is mentally strong and positive, and even the worst misfortune failed to drag him down from a cheerful and calm state of mind.

Broken Toys Cannot Make You Unhappy

Let's look at little children again, for example. If their toys are broken, they cry for a while and then start playing again. They don't live in that bad state forever, unlike adults, who brood over the same thoughts again and again for days, months, or years. Children are the epitome of joyful and cheerful living. No matter what happens around them, they have a knack for putting themselves back into a happy mood. Do you notice how easily they do it? They don't think much about how to do it—they just do it! Then, could it be true that joy is our natural state of mind? Could it be that we don't have to learn anything to be happy? Could it be that we don't really need anything external to find peace of mind?

Thinking logically, the answer seems to be *yes*. Little kids don't think a lot about being happy. They just are happy! We all step out of that natural state of happiness once in a while into an unhappy state of mind. With kids, it's very transient. However, as you grow into an adult, you spend a lot of time in that unhappy state of mind—it's called *stress. We use the power of our thinking against ourselves and get locked up in a stressful state of mind.*

> We use the power of our thinking against ourselves and get locked up in a stressful state of mind.

Why Are You Still Unhappy Even After Your Basic Needs Are Fulfilled?

We limit our happiness to certain conditions. *The deeper you get buried in conditional happiness and the more conditions you need to be happy, the harder it is for you to be happy.* Think about this logically . . . it makes sense. If you want ten cars before you can be happy, the likelihood of you being happy is much less than a person who is happy with just one car. You might ask, "What about my needs?" Yes, of course, your basic needs must be fulfilled. Most of us have fulfilled our basic needs, and have achieved much beyond that, but we still are stressed in our lives. If not, why would there be so many doctors, celebrities, attorneys, businesspeople, and others with lots of money, fame, fans, and possessions who are still stressed, depressed, unhappy, and even suicidal? It's because they strayed far

> The deeper you get buried in conditional happiness and the more conditions you need to be happy, the harder it is for you to be happy.

away from their natural and happy state of mind to an abnormal state of distress, mistaking transient pleasures for true happiness. Remember, though, even if your pendulum of balance has drifted far from normal, if you allow it to, it can swing back right away and rebalance itself. *That is the power of resilience.*

DR. CALM'S PRESCRIPTION

1 Life is a series of challenges; that's the nature of life. No matter whether you are rich or poor, healthy or unhealthy, Black or White, we all have our own challenges to face.

2 *Resiliency* is your capacity to heal, your capacity to be flexible with life, your capacity to recalibrate yourself and reclaim your lost joy, peace, and contentment in life. *Resiliency* is your capacity to revert from a stressful state of mind to a calm state of mind.

3 No matter what your situation is, and no matter how deep you are buried in troubles, know that you have the innate capacity to bounce back. That capacity is called *resiliency*, which is the indomitable nature of the human spirit.

4 Your ability to be emotionally resilient is independent of your social status, color, creed, race, religion, money, your past, or any other limiting condition.

5 The difference between those who succeed versus those who struggle: Those who are successful have used their innate power of resilience to overcome their challenges, and those who struggle, either knowingly or unknowingly, haven't tapped into that power.

6 Know that the power of resilience within you is never lacking and is never broken.

7 When you exercise your power of resilience daily, it eventually leads to such strength that you literally become stress resistant, where nothing can ruffle you.

Stress — The Health Epidemic of the 21st Century

Part II Objectives

- Identify the dangers of stress in relation to your health, happiness, relationships, finances, and other aspects of life.
- Recognize that stress breeds antisocial elements and terrorism.
- Know that eliminating stress results in happier and healthier individuals, families, and societies.

CHAPTER 3

The Seven Deadly Consequences of Stress

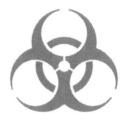

Stress is a silent killer. Don't ignore it.

The Unspoken Truth About Stress

Stress is a global epidemic according to the United Nations. The World Health Organization defines stress as *the* health epidemic of the 21st century. I go a little further and say stress is the biggest epidemic in the history of the world. No epidemic has affected as many people in the world as stress does. Plague killed around 100 million people in 541–542 A.D. and 50 million in

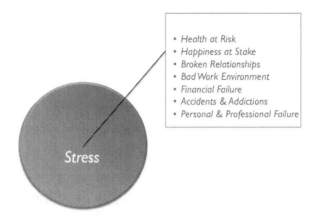

- *Health at Risk*
- *Happiness at Stake*
- *Broken Relationships*
- *Bad Work Environment*
- *Financial Failure*
- *Accidents & Addictions*
- *Personal & Professional Failure*

Stress

Figure 3.1. The Seven Deadly Consequences of Stress

1346–1350 A.D. It was called Black Death at that time. The great influenza pandemic affected 50 to 100 million people in 1918. HIV/AIDS has affected 40 million people so far since 1960s. Put together, the number of people who suffer from these and many other epidemics like malaria, cholera, tuberculosis, etc., is less than half a billion people. Now compare that with the number of people who are stressed every day. Look at any set of health statistics. At least half of the world population, 3.75 billion, is stressed at any point of time. That's being very conservative. The real numbers are probably much higher, possibly close to 70–75 percent. That's almost three-quarters (5.7 billion) of the world's population (7.6 billion as of October 2017). That number is astounding!

When was the last time any epidemic has affected so many people? Then why is it not getting the amount of attention and resources needed? It is because *stress is an invisible epidemic. It's a slow and silent killer,* unlike plague, flu, or cholera, which cause dramatic death in a short period of time. Stress is the *elephant in room,* being ignored completely. Neither the government, the medical establishment, the school or social system has properly

Stress is an invisible epidemic. It's a slow and silent killer.

addressed this New Age epidemic. The result is most people have no formal or even informal stress management training; they do not know how to manage their stress, let alone prevent it. The world as a whole has failed miserably in tackling this gigantic problem of the 21st century.

It is a well-known fact that chronic stress results in many diseases and illnesses. In fact, chronic stress is the foundation that most chronic illnesses build upon. To just get a glimpse of the harmful effects of stress in your life, see the next section. My intention in sharing this information is not to scare you but to educate you about the importance of living a stress-free life.

The Seven Deadly Consequences of Stress (see Figure 3.1.)

Stress is directly or indirectly related to all the following problems:

1. Your physical health is at risk of

- Heart attack
- Stroke
- Cancer
- Cirrhosis
- Fibromyalgia and more

2. Mental anguish and unhappiness is the source of

- Anxiety
- Worry
- Depression
- Suicide
- Post-traumatic stress disorder and more

3. Stressed relationships can lead to

- Misunderstandings
- Anger and resentment toward self and others
- Conflict with friends and family

- Divorce
- Abuse and more

4. High stress at work can result in

- Absenteeism (both body and mind absent)
- "Presenteeism" (body present but mind absent)
- Poor performance
- Communication failure
- Rifts between you (the employee) and management

5. A stressed mind is prone to dangerous behaviors such as

- Accidents, because you are distracted, behaving irritably, and making hasty decisions
- Addictions, which are incorrect coping mechanisms used as a method of escape from stress that include using and abusing alcohol, drugs, and smoking

6. Stress leads to financial failure because

- Your attention is scattered and thus your energies are wasted
- You feel tired and inefficient
- Your poor decision-making results in poor money management
- You're squandering money as a method of escape from stress
- You are "stress shopping"

7. You might experience personal and professional failure because

- You've lost your focus and direction in life
- You're confused about your true identity and purpose in life
- You feel disconnected from nature, yourself, and the Higher Power
- Frustration becomes a part of your life
- The end result of relentless stress is often total failure in life

One of my fellow physicians shared the following story with me, and it underscores the importance of living a stress-free life.

I was at the airport, sitting on a chair and working on my laptop, waiting for the connecting flight. That place was very noisy, but I was totally focused on what I was doing. Usually, when I am intently working on something, my brain filters out all the noise and disturbances around me, but this time I was distracted by a man's loud, intrusive voice shouting over the phone almost twenty feet away. I lifted my head and looked to my left in his direction. I noticed that other people had also taken notice. Some were amused by his behavior, some had scornful expressions, and some were disturbed by the entire situation.

I looked more closely at the man who was causing this ruckus. He was a Caucasian man in his late forties, medium height and build, wearing a navy-blue suit and tie, a Bluetooth earpiece, and shouting over the phone, seemingly unaware of his surroundings. I could not completely comprehend his conversation, but I could see that he was desperate for something. He was trying to conduct a business transaction, and it seemed like things were not going well for him. This went on for almost fifteen minutes.

Suddenly, he dropped his phone, tightly clutched his chest, and collapsed onto the floor. Everyone around him, alerted by this emergency, ran toward and reached out to him. I threw my laptop into my bag and quickly ran over too to see if I could be of any medical help. He looked pale and seemed short of breath with his face contorted in pain, which are typical symptoms of chest pain due to a heart attack. I felt his pulse and was relieved to feel it strong; he did not lose consciousness. That gave me a chance to quickly ask a few questions to confirm my suspicion. This was an obvious medical emergency. Ambulance and emergency medical personnel were called right away. Help arrived within a few minutes. He was given oxygen via an oxygen mask and some aspirin and nitroglycerin, and he was taken away to the nearest hospital. I felt relieved and hoped for the best for him, although I do not know the outcome.

Did you notice how this person developed a heart attack because of his emotional outburst? It is well known in the medical community that stress can precipitate heart disease and many other health problems. I see that all the time in my patients. The good news is we can prevent stress and related health problems by practicing calmness. New research suggests that people who are calm and relaxed have fewer heart problems and their blood pressure improves with meditation, sometimes even without medication. The American Heart Association recommends meditation and relaxation techniques to reduce blood pressure and heart disease.

If stress does not affect your body in any way, then you might not care. But, unfortunately, stress affects both your body and mind. As a physician, I have seen many patients with strong minds and positive outlooks on life suffer less and recover faster from illness. On the contrary, people who are stressed tend to have more severe physical symptoms for a prolonged period, and they magnify their suffering because of their negative state of mind. To my stressed patients, I give simple relaxation exercises to calm them down immediately, and the moment they calm down, they feel better. Their blood pressure improves, their blood glucose improves, and they start feeling more positive about their upcoming procedure. Such is the impact of your mind on your physical and mental well-being.

Consequence 1: Stress Jeopardizes Your Physical Health

Stress is linked to the five leading causes of death in the United States:

1. Heart disease
2. Cancer
3. Lung disease
4. Accidents (unintentional injuries)
5. Stroke

Stress adversely affects the human body in many ways. When we are stressed, our blood vessels constrict, leading to a reduced supply of blood and nutrients to the tissues, which results in pain and poorly functioning organs. This can be easily demonstrated by muscle pain that is caused by *trigger points*, which are *hyperalgesic* (overly painful) and hyperirritable knots in our muscles and *fascia* (a band or sheet of connective tissue, primarily collagen, beneath the skin that attaches, stabilizes, encloses, and separates muscles and other internal organs). These trigger points are very sensitive to pain stimuli. People who suffer from back pain and muscle tightness often have these trigger points in their bodies whether they are aware of them or not. Stress is one of the key factors contributing to the development of trigger points, muscle aches, back pain, and fibromyalgia (a medical condition characterized by chronic widespread pain and a heightened pain response to pressure).

Muscles tighten because of stress and poor circulation. Tightness and pain lead to less mobility and the accumulation of toxins. The toxins are not cleared from the body because of poor circulation. This, again, stimulates another cycle of tightness, less motion, and more pain. More trigger points will be formed. This can become a self-perpetuating phenomenon unless the stress cycle is interrupted. When you go to a physical therapist or trigger point specialist, the specialist will work on those points and try to mobilize them to increase blood circulation so that these points relax and resolve themselves. Often, relaxation techniques that reduce your stress levels also help to relieve these trigger points.

A heart attack is another major health consequence of stress. Most of us unfortunately have probably had the real-life experience of witnessing or hearing about a highly stressed person all of a sudden suffering a heart attack or stroke. In fact, there is a variant of heart attack caused purely by emotional distress. When the doctor performs a procedure called *coronary angiogram* and looks at such a patient's blood vessels (in the heart), everything looks normal because the constricted blood vessels causing the chest pain have already relaxed by then. This is called *vasospastic angina* (spasm of blood vessels in the heart) in medical terms.

The list of harmful effects of stress on your body is endless. Stress digs deeper than you think.

1. Stress makes your blood stickier, thus increasing the risk of clots forming in your legs and lungs.
2. Chronic stress triggers inflammation, which is the common denominator for many chronic diseases.
3. Stress degrades your immune system, making you more susceptible to infections. Men who are HIV-positive who are stressed are more prone to advance to AIDS infection than those who are not stressed.
4. Stressed people tend to have poor blood pressure and diabetes control.
5. Stress can trigger headaches, migraines, neck pain, and back pain.

So, the take home point is this: If you want to experience good health, keep stress at bay.

Consequence 2: A Stressed Mind Makes More Mistakes

When you are stressed, your thinking becomes muddled, you can't discern good from bad, your judgment is impaired, and you make wrong decisions and act hastily. This leads to unnecessary mistakes and complications, which, in turn, lead to more stress. When you are stressed, good thoughts and solutions do not come to mind. I can't emphasize enough how important it is to remain calm regardless of the circumstances. I have noticed many times in my own life and in the lives of others how things fall into place when the mind is calm and relaxed.

Recently, in a seminar I conducted, one of the attendees shared this experience and graciously granted permission to use this example in this book. (For the sake of privacy, I have not used her real name.)

One day, Julie was going from work to her 2 p.m. doctor's appointment. Because of the inefficiencies of a high stress job, she was late to finish the tasks at hand. It's already past 2 p.m.! She rushed from her office, got into the car, and hastily drove to her doctor's office. She wanted to call the doctor's office about the delay, and as she searched her handbag, she quickly realized that she had left her cell phone on the desk in her office. Her phone contained important personal information that she couldn't afford anyone to see. She was anxious about it.

As her mind was preoccupied with the thoughts about her cell phone, she missed an exit. Now she had to turn around and take a longer route, which further delayed her trip. Because she was getting even later for her appointment, she started speeding at 90 mph. A police officer appeared out of nowhere, as if just waiting for this moment. She tried to explain the situation, but the officer would not listen to her. But what was even more frustrating was that it took a ridiculously long amount of time for him to record all the information on her driver's license, even in this high-tech world!

After much aggravation, she finally reached her doctor's office, but as she looked at her watch, she noticed that she was late to her appointment by almost an hour! As she apologized, the doctor's secretary absolutely surprised her by saying, "It's alright. Doc is running behind schedule today. We will accommodate you!" With a sigh of great relief, she thought, "All this time I worried unnecessarily, missed the exit, forgot my phone, had to pay $200 for speeding, and got points on my driving license. All the anxiety I went through was really not worth it!"

This experience prompted her to wholeheartedly apply the Principles she had learned from my seminar. Julie was excited to see that these Principles are practical and produce positive results in life. She was happy because she was not missing any more doctor's appointments and has been more efficient at work; therefore, she can leave work earlier and have more time for her kids and family. Everyone around her started seeing her as a calm person who they could seek counsel from instead of viewing her as a Nervous Nellie.

Moral of the story: *If you want a smooth ride in life, make sure to maintain a calm mind!*

Consequence 3: Stressed Relationships at Home Lead to Divorce and At-Risk Children

When there is stress in a marital relationship, the wife and husband will be less understanding of each other. Without true understanding, love cannot flourish. Without love, there will be no empathy. Without empathy, there is no humanity. Without humanity, relationships perish. In a marriage, that might lead to separation and divorce (see Figure 3.2).

When parents are stressed, they will be consumed by their own problems and pay less attention to their kids. As a result, children may look for attention from outsiders. If they fall in with bad company, they may develop bad habits, even addictions (see Figure 3.3). Often, when kids have strong parental love, attention, and support, they feel less peer pressure. That is why—on behalf of all our wonderful children—we should keep stress out of our lives so that they can have a bright and promising future.

Stressed Relationship Between Wife & Husband: Risk of Divorce

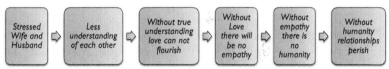

Figure 3.2. Stressed Relationship Between Wife and Husband

Poor Family Dynamics: Kids Gone Wrong

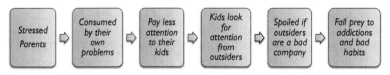

Figure 3.3. Stressed Family and its Bad Effects on Children

Consequence 4: Stress at Workplace leads to Poor Performance and Ailing Organizations

A stressed boss is a menace at work. Stressed bosses tend to be less supportive and more judgmental. He or she will be less appreciative of others' efforts and ignorant of the perspectives of the employees. This leads to conflict; consideration and compassion go out of window. The result is an unhappy and disgruntled employee.

After multiple failed attempts to win the praise of a stressed boss, an unhappy and disgruntled employee will finally resort to a lackadaisical attitude and adopt a passive work ethic. He or she will just do the bare minimum to get the work done, will find another job, or open a part-time business which will deprive the company of the most important resource—an employee's time, undivided attention, whole-hearted effort, and commitment to the excellence and growth of the organization.

That's why it is extremely important to train your managers and executives to be stress-free.

Once they are calm and composed, all leadership and managerial skills they learned will be of use. Otherwise all those skills will not get a chance to be put into practical application, which would help you run your organization smoothly and the company's performance will sky rocket.

Employees, when stressed for any reason, whether work related or personal life related, do not perform well. They will be frequently absent from work (absenteeism) and if they do show up, their bodies are present, but minds are absent (presenteeism). You need to identify them and help them early on before you lose them completely.

A powerful elephant with a sharp nail in its foot won't be able to walk. So, it won't be able to find food and nourish itself. It will eventually die of hunger and thirst. In a similar way, *even the most powerful and highly skilled workers in your organization can't perform well if they are stressed.* The nail in the foot can be compared to the stress in an employee's life. Identify them early and help them. The cost of implementing a stress management program is much less than hiring another employee and training someone again.

NIOSH, the National Institute of Occupational Safety and Health recommends workplace stress intervention for healthy and productive employees. Make sure you have one at your organization.

Consequence 5: Stress Triggers Risky Behaviors and Addictions

Stress affects your behavior, too. When stressed, you tend to be more defensive and not listen to the wise counsel of friends, family, and colleagues. When stressed, your mind becomes irritable, impulsive, and reactive. Reason flies out the window. In that state of mind, you are more accident prone and are likely to be involved in high-risk behaviors.

Often, to escape from stress, you adopt unhealthy behaviors. You develop poor coping mechanisms and may indulge in harmful habits, such as smoking, drinking, or doing drugs, which provide a temporary, pseudo-escape from stress but ultimately are detrimental to your health. Moreover, the power of addiction can enslave you, and soon you will find yourself deep in the grips of disease and death.

The P-E-T System for Stress-Free Living will help you avoid such pseudo-pleasures in the first place. If you are naturally joyful and peaceful, you won't be easily attracted to pseudo-pleasures and addictions; in fact, you will develop a natural aversion to them and will be inclined to choose healthy behaviors instead.

Consequence 6: Stress Shopping and Financial Failure

Do you know people in your circle of family members, friends, and colleagues who go on a shopping spree whenever they are stressed and buy new clothes or something else only to find that their partner is not happy with this behavior? Then they argue and add more stress to their life. I know many people like that. When you are in the grip of stress you tend to squander money easily. You feel money will make up for the peace of mind and happiness you lack. So, you go on a shopping spree hoping to find happiness in that new beautiful watch, an expensive handbag, an exotic car, or a huge home, failing to recognize that no amount of external possessions can fill the void you feel within. Stress shopping can quickly bankrupt even the richest people on the earth. There are too many expensive toys in this world that can drain all your money in no time. There are many celebrities and sports stars who became penniless because of stress shopping and poor financial decisions. Average people like us have no chance to survive it.

This era of online shopping created the most perfect conditions for bankruptcy-made-easy. Previously you had to make the effort to go to a mall or a store to buy something. Now, just with the click of a mouse you can lose thousands of dollars. Literally, you could order anything you want on Amazon, eBay, Apple, and many other online stores. That's quite unfortunate. Though online shopping is convenient and has its advantages, you must be ever watchful not to get addicted to it. Also, stressed people tend to make poor decisions and costly mistakes leading to disastrous financial consequences. *So, if you want to be financially savvy, be stress savvy first.*

Consequence 7: Stress Leads to Personal and Professional Failure

When you are stressed, you make mistakes. Mistakes may lead to lowered self-confidence and, over time, low self-esteem. If you have low self-esteem, you can be easily taken advantage of in our society. You might settle for less-than-good relationships, be abused, or experience mistreatment. This can trigger depression or other psychiatric problems. You can develop poor sleep patterns. You might feel alienated and become fearful of almost everything. Because of this fear and doubt, you refuse help even when offered in the spirit of goodwill. You feel disconnected from yourself, nature, and the Higher Power. Confusion reigns within and without. You may fall prey to addictions. Slowly, your overall quality of life slips. Ultimately, you might commit suicide or become antisocial and dangerous. I hope no one reaches this very dangerous stage of life. *Unfortunately, there are many people who attempt suicide each day. Life, once gone, cannot be brought back.* If you see anyone who is in dire need and under great stress, help them in any way you can.

Stress and Mental Health Problems in Society

The effects of stress do not end at a personal level. Stress invariably affects the people around you, whether they are colleagues, friends, or loved ones both near and far. *Personal stress slowly becomes interpersonal and societal.* Stress creeps into your relationships at work and home. You lose work–life balance.

How often do you hear about some horrible incident like shootings in public places like schools, restaurants, and shopping malls? It happens way too often! These incidents are actually extreme forms of stress. If stressed people are not identified early (hopefully as early as in their childhood

> Personal stress slowly becomes interpersonal and societal.

or young adulthood), their unhappiness and negativity can rapidly bloom, and then be released (like toxic pollen) in a dangerous form of mental illness called terrorism and violence (see Figure 3.4).

Terrorism—The Most Evil Outcome of Stress

Look at the world around you. The whole world is going through hell! See how many terrorist attacks happened in the

A Stressed Mind is the Devil's Workshop

For our own existence and for the sustainment of a good society, it is vital that we address stress both at work and home before it breeds anti-social elements in society

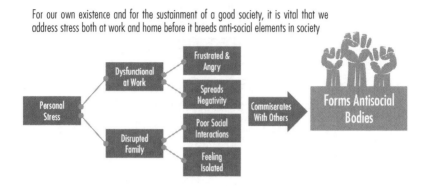

Figure 3.4. Stress Leads to Terrorism

recent past! You have seen the evil extremist groups like ISIS beheading people and, even worse, posting the pictures on the Internet as if the killing was the greatest accomplishment in human history. Look at the attacks in Paris in November 2015 where hundreds were held hostage and ruthlessly killed. How about the terrorist attacks on Brussels in Belgium, Manchester and London in the United Kingdom, San Bernardino in the United States, Istanbul in Turkey, and many other countries? How about the Syrian crisis? How many innocent children, men, and women were killed because of terrorism in the past year? How many families were devastated because of such ruthless terrorist acts? How much of our property and financial resources are being destroyed every year because of terrorism? How much money is being spent to fight terrorism? Billions, if not trillions, of dollars. *The root cause of all this terrorism is **stress**.* Yes, it's true. It's stress! When people are unhappy and stressed, they do bad things. And stress begets stress!

It's About Time to Dedicate More Resources to Anti-Stress Efforts

Looking at all these dangers of stress, we can no longer view stress as a simple problem at a personal level. We must recognize the dangers of stress both at a personal and societal level. Much money is being spent on the aftermath of stress, creating financial burdens throughout society—on our health care industry for the care of chronic disease; on our social system because of poor relationships, divorces, and lawsuits; on our workplaces because of poor organizational productivity due to absenteeism and stress-related problems; and so on. *It's important that we take the stress monster seriously and collectively defeat it and reestablish peace and harmony in our families and society.*

It's important that we take the stress monster seriously and collectively defeat it and reestablish peace and harmony in our families and society.

DR. CALM'S PRESCRIPTION

1   Know that stress is a silent killer. Don't fall prey to it.

2   Stress is associated with five leading causes of death, including heart attacks, cancer, and strokes. So, do not risk your health by ignoring stress.

3   Unhappy relationships are a major source of stress for people in all walks of life. Poor relationships lead to poor family dynamics and stressful work environment. Resolve the stress in your relationships.

4   Parental stress has a strong impact on children's well-being. Do not let your stress destroy your children's lives. If you think your relationship with your spouse is adversely affecting your children, do not wait any longer—stop and fix that problem first.

5   If you are an employer or a manager, know that workplace stress can destroy your company's performance and your employees' motivation. Stressed employees call in sick often, make errors, or get into accidents posing danger to self and others. Make sure your organization has an employee stress relief program.

6   Stressed people tend to "stress shop" and squander their money. Their energies are scattered, they feel tired, and they make poor financial decisions, resulting in bankruptcy. So, keep calm and be financially savvy.

7   Many people resort to poor coping mechanisms like drinking alcohol, smoking, or doing drugs when stressed. Know that addictions do not relieve stress; they temporarily mask it until the problems in your life consume you. Do not fall into this dangerous trap.

CHAPTER 4

The Ubiquitous Nature of Stress

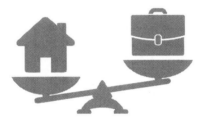

Professional and personal stress are not two separate entities.
They are different manifestations of the same stress.

The Brutality of Life

My life sucks. My wife hates me. We don't get along at all. I can't come out of the relationship. There is too much at stake. It will badly affect my children's well-being. I made many attempts to right our relationship but each time it lasts a few days and then falls apart again. I don't know what to do. I am afraid if we continue like this, one of us will die of stress. Or get admitted to a psychiatric hospital.

This job is killing me. I work long hours, and I'm not earning enough. My boss is a menace at work. He just doesn't understand our problems. My talents are not recognized at all. If he openheartedly embraces me, I can work wonders. But I know that's not going to happen. His ego is too big to appreciate others' efforts. How do I turn around this situation? I need help!!!

My husband is very sick. I am the only caregiver and the breadwinner for the family. I am distressed constantly. I worry about the future of our family. I fear for my husband's life. I can't keep my thoughts under control. My mind becomes foggy. I feel tired. I am afraid I am going to make a big mistake at work and risk losing my job. How do I calm down and get a handle over my life situation?

I am the CEO of a Fortune 500 company. I make lot of money. But I am deeply unhappy. I don't know why. Why don't all the money, possessions, and pleasures give me lasting happiness? Why do I feel a void within? What should I do to find true and lasting happiness? I will give you all that I have if you can show me a way out!

I am a nurse manager. I manage a whole floor in the hospital. My nurses think my job is easy. They feel that I am bossing around and doing nothing. They have no clue! This managerial role is taking a toll on me. There are too many deadlines, too much to do, and too many demands from the administration. I can't do it anymore. I am losing my sanity. How can I multitask? How can I perform under pressure?

I am a doctor. Everyone thinks doctors' lives are enviable and we all have lots of money, social status, expensive cars, and large homes. People have no idea how difficult our lives are. Doctors die early. We are at great risk of depression and suicide. We don't have time to take care of ourselves. We're always busy! We have lost our autonomy to large health organizations and insurance companies, who make all rules. We have little control over our life. It is the Washington lobbyists and attorneys who control our health care system. I just feel like a puppet. How can I practice peacefully in this dysfunctional health care system? How can I fulfill my duties to my patients without worrying that I will be sued?

I want to change the world. There is way too much suffering in this world. I feel the pain of many who are suffering because of lack of food, drinking water, and basic facilities. There is too much dying because of disease and famine in the poor parts of the world. But I have a career that prevents me from traveling around the world and helping people. How do I find a way to balance my life by doing service to people and achieve financial stability?

I lost my job. Suddenly, I received the termination letter from my employer and my future is dire. I can't believe it. How do I find hope and strength during these difficult times? Will I find another job? How do I do that? My mind is restless, and I can't focus on anything. Can you help me?

———————

Something terrible happened in my life. My husband and our 12-year-old son went to the mall the other day. A crazy person opened fire and started shooting people. I lost my child and my husband was deeply injured. I trembled with fear. I can't get over the sorrow of my loss. How can I console myself? I don't feel like living anymore. I am afraid to send my other child to school or anywhere outside home. What do I do?

———————

I am moody and emotional. I tried many times to not be emotional, but I can't help it. Little things bother me easily and drag me down to bad mood. I know my moodiness is badly affecting my relationships both at work and home. I feel like I am a slave to my emotions. How do I overcome moodiness? How can I become emotionally stable?

All these are deeply painful true-life situations representing how brutal life can sometimes be. The stress people are experiencing in these situations is paramount and sometimes paralyzing. I understand how painful it can be when you are caught up in those kinds of situations. I truly do! I tried to address most of these problems in this book, in one way or another. I want to reassure you that there are solutions to your problems. There is hope. There is light at the end of tunnel. Be patient. Don't lose faith. Keep reading this book and you will gain new insights that show solutions to your problems. I have made the advice practical and easy to apply to your life now!

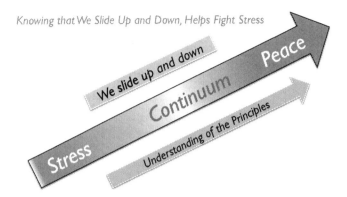

Figure 4.1. We Slide Up and Down the Stress–Peace Continuum

To Stress is Human

Occasionally, we all feel stressed. That's normal for us as human beings. But to live in a stressful state every day is abnormal and harmful to you and the people around you. We all live on a stress–peace continuum in life. We all go in and out of stress. In Figure 4.1, you see that at one end of the stress–peace continuum there is extreme stress and at the other end there is boundless peace. We all slide up and down on this stress–peace continuum. The greater your understanding of the Three Principles, the better your chances are to stay on the peaceful side of this continuum. If you are ignorant of these Principles, the chances are high that you will spend most of your time on the stressful side of this continuum.

Stress Is Ubiquitous and Has No Boundaries

Stress in your personal life overflows into your professional life and vice versa. Sometimes, you feel so tired at work that you can barely perform the tasks at hand. After a busy day, you often go to sleep thinking about the problems you have at work with your boss, the deadlines you must meet, or something else that's bothering you. These thoughts interfere with your sleep. You wake up feeling tired, restless, and irritable. Not a great way to start the day! Your day begins with stress even before you fully wake up! And so, the stress cycle continues.

> Stress is all-pervasive; stress has no boundaries. It does not respect time and space.

Stress is all-pervasive; stress has no boundaries. It does not respect time and space. If unchecked, stress during the day will be carried into the night, and vice versa. The stress you have in the morning spills over into the afternoon and persists through the evening and stays with you through the following night. You won't sleep well. The same stress will encroach into your next day if you don't stay determined to remain calm.

Are You Righteously Miserable?

No matter what the reason is, it doesn't help to get upset and lose your temper. That's true even if you have all the right reasons for getting upset! So, don't lose your cool! *Come what may, do what you must do from a calm state of mind.* In the following situation, notice that as soon as I became calm, I started seeing solutions for my problems and got out of trouble. The external events started losing their impact on me. Things started rolling along well. That's the power of a calm mind.

I still remember the morning when I was very upset with a company from which I had bought a laptop. A few days after I bought it, it crashed. It had some kind of malfunction. I called customer service. After being put on hold for a long time, I was able to reach a customer service representative. After being asked a lot of questions in a 20-minute conversation, he transferred me to another department that was supposed to take care of the issue.

Once I was transferred, the second representative started all over from the beginning, asking me the same irritating questions. I explained the problem again. After listening, the representative said he couldn't really help because of a sub-clause written in its policy (the fine print that's written in tiny letters that you need a magnifying glass to read). I did not agree with him because I knew that the reason for the malfunction in the computer was not my fault. So, I asked him to transfer me to the manager. Now, after explaining the situation for the third time to the manager, who was rude to begin with and who did not want to investigate the problem, I started losing my temper. After a hot-tempered discussion, I hung up.

I felt deceived and taken advantage of by this company. Meanwhile, I realized that it was getting late and I had to go work. I quickly walked down the stairs, entered the garage, got into my car, and hastily drove out of the driveway. Within 200 feet, I was at an intersection but failed to notice another car driving through it. By the time I realized what was going on, the other car had hit me. If I were calm, I would have noticed that car and would have avoided the accident. But I was upset, and my mind was clouded with bad feelings. So I failed to notice the other car; it was as if there had been a blind spot in my eye. On top of everything, because I was angry, I was driving faster than usual. The end result was I got into an accident.

Once I realized what had happened, I immediately got out of my car and saw a young woman. She stopped her car. She was safe and not hurt but was crying hysterically. As I consoled her and turned back toward my car, I noticed my rear bumper was dented and broken. That made me even more upset. It was going to cost me dearly to replace it. But I had no time to think about that. I was already very late for work and was worried about my waiting patients.

I called the auto insurance company and went through the normal drill. I was thinking, If my insurance does not cover this, it will cost me a lot for the repair. I was worried about it. I got to work very late and was very stressed. I labored to finish my day and arrived home late at night, completely drained. I could not sleep well that night because of the restless thoughts storming my mind: the laptop that was not working, the broken rear bumper of my car and whether it was covered by insurance, whether I would have to shell out a fortune out of my own pocket to fix my car, and the possibility of an increased insurance premium as a result.

However, the next morning when I woke up, I made a firm decision: Whatever happens, I am not going to let those thoughts bother me. I needed to put myself back into a good state of mind. The fact that I was righteously upset and angry was not going to help my situation. It was only going to make the situation worse. Then why should I stress? After all, I have a choice. I do not have to react to the situation and I can choose my response wisely. So, I put into action *The PET System of Stress-Free Living* and guess what happened? I calmed down! All the restless thoughts came to an abrupt halt. I was back in a good mood. I accepted things as they were and went with the flow for the rest of the day.

The next day, I received a call from the auto insurance

company and was told that it would cover the accident with a deductible. They would consider it as a no-fault accident. I couldn't believe it. I felt so happy. Hurray! My insurance premium wouldn't go up. In that happy state of mind, all of a sudden, I also realized that even though the company that I had bought my laptop from did not want to rectify its mistake, the credit card that I had purchased the laptop with had an extended warranty plan for up to a year. I called the issuer and it honored the warranty. In the end, everything magically fell into place. I emerged from the situation unscathed but learned a powerful lesson. 'No matter how bad your situation might look like, never lose your cool.'

You see how stress has no respect for your time? It will consume all your time, if unchecked. If not for your innate ability to halt restless thoughts and become calm and relaxed, stress marches on, leading to other bad events in your life. Sometimes, you see people like that: something bad has happened, and they carry the weight of that stress for many days and weeks. You must learn how to break away from the stress cycle or you are at great risk of losing happiness, money, relationships, health, and more.

What's the point of harboring anger, resentment, or other negative emotions in your heart? It does not help anyone, and it certainly does not help you. Being irritated for every little reason drains your energy. People will avoid you. No one wants to be around someone who is constantly irritable and upset.

But there are people in this world who are cool and calm regardless of the circumstances. These people know that getting stressed is not going to help anyone, including themselves. Surrounding yourself with such people will elevate your emotional well-being by instilling calmness, confidence, and positive feelings.

DR. CALM'S PRESCRIPTION

1 ✓ Although life is beautiful, there are times when it can be absolutely brutal. Stay put. There is hope. There is always light at the end of tunnel.

2 ✓ Unfortunately, stress is as ubiquitous as bacteria and viruses. Even bacteria and viruses undergo stress. But, know that most stress in life is preventable if you follow the right principles and techniques.

3 ✓ Professional stress and personal stress are not two separate entities. They are interrelated. Stress at home affects your work performance, and workplace stress encroaches into your personal life. Try not to carry your personal stress to work, and vice versa.

4 ✓ Regardless of the place, circumstance, and reason, losing your cool doesn't help. Keep calm and carry on.

5 ✓ Acknowledge that to stress once in a while is normal and part of being human; however, to get stressed frequently and remain there for long periods is abnormal.

6 ✓ We all live on a stress–peace continuum, and we slide up and down on it. The goal of life is to stay on the peaceful side of this spectrum more and more.

7 ✓ Developing resilience and internal resistance to external challenges is the cornerstone for stress prevention and management. One day, you will become so strong emotionally that you will stand unshaken amid crashing worlds.

Understanding Stress and Debunking the Myths

Part III Objectives

- Learn the true definition of stress.
- Debunk the myths about stress.
- Uncover the real source of stress in your life.
- Escape the iron grip of stressors.
- Differentiate acute stress from chronic stress.
- Tap into the power of your rational brain.
- Check your stress levels.

CHAPTER 5

The Ten Costly Myths about Stress

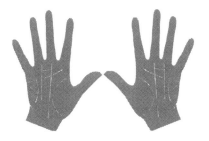

Your destiny depends on your ability to differentiate truth from myth.

The Power of Myth

People believed for thousands of years that Earth was flat and the center of the universe until Copernicus, Plato, and other brave astronomers and philosophers yelled out, "Hey! Earth is round like a sphere! The Sun is the center of our solar system, and the Earth revolves around the Sun and not the other way around!"

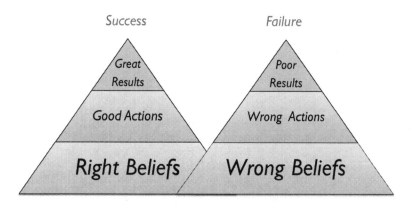

Figure 5.1. Beliefs vs. Success

For a moment, just imagine if we had continued to believe that Earth was flat and the center of the universe: all the astronomical calculations by our scientists would have been utterly wrong. Human civilization would not have scientifically progressed this far. We could not have learned how to send satellites into space, get information about our planet, obtain details about the weather, create GPS capabilities, and so on. We would probably not have television, radio, the Internet, and many other modern gadgets. Can you imagine life without the Internet, cell phones, movies, and your favorite television shows? Ugh! Most boring!! It would be like going back to the Stone Age. We definitely don't want that . . . right?

Do you see how one seemingly true but profoundly wrong belief could adversely affect the face of humanity and all the innovations on Earth? In the same way, your wrong beliefs about stress prevent you from living a peaceful and joyful life.

Your Beliefs Determine Your Success

Belief is the foundation of our thoughts and actions. If you base your actions on misconceptions and wrong beliefs, you are doomed to fail, no matter how hard you try to succeed. If you base your actions on truth, you progress and prosper (see Figure 5.1).

While you can make commitments and resolutions to live a stress-free life, you will not succeed until you acquire the right knowledge toward attaining stress freedom and put that in action. Unfortunately, most people have false beliefs about stress. Those false beliefs can prove costly, as they may spend all their resources and their whole life based on those wrong beliefs. Your efforts based on these false ideas will not relieve stress, but, in fact, might worsen it. First, debunk the myths and automatically you will make progress.

> If you base your actions on misconceptions and wrong beliefs, you are doomed to fail, no matter how hard you try to succeed.

The next section discusses ten costly myths about stress. As you move forward in the book, these myths will dissolve one by one, and leave you with a true understanding of what underlies a peaceful and joyful life—and how you can experience it!

Myth #1 Stress is out there and is the result of external circumstances.

Truth #1 Stress happens within. While external events do have some influence on us, it is our response to them that finally determines if we get stressed or not.

Myth #2 There is no way out of stress, and we must succumb to it.

Truth #2 Stress is an illusion created through our thoughts. We are the thinkers of our thoughts. The moment we realize that, we will stop misusing our thoughts, and all stress disappears.

Myth #3 Being stressed means you are successful.

Truth #3 Success has no meaning if you are stressed and not happy with yourself. Real success is a measure of peace of mind in balance with abundance.

Myth #4 No symptoms mean not stressed.

Truth #4 Symptoms of stress are just the tip of the iceberg. Many people do not have symptoms, or they are not aware of the symptoms they have. So, they think that they are not stressed. Most people have chronic stress in their lives that adversely affects their health and relationships.

Myth #5 Alcohol, tobacco, and drugs reduce our stress.

Truth #5 They don't. Alcohol, tobacco, and drugs give you a feeling of elation or sedation, letting you ignore the cause of stress in your life and mask the real problems that grow like cancer within.

Myth #6 Someone pushes our buttons.

Truth #6 No one can push our buttons. You are bothered by others only to the extent you allow others to bother you, because of your own inner vulnerabilities.

Myth #7 Some stress is needed to stay motivated and be productive.

Truth #7 Incessant stress makes you feel tired, less motivated, and less productive. All human beings are endowed with an innate spark that motivates them to grow, contribute, and create. That is what motivates you. A calm mind facilitates all inspiration, creativity, and productivity.

Myth #8 It is okay to ignore stress as long as there are no immediate problems.

Truth#8 Do not ignore stress. Stress ignored over time is detrimental to your health and happiness. Preventing stress is easier and better than managing it.

Myth #9 A little stress is okay in life.

Truth #9 No stress is necessary in life because stress begets stress.

Myth #10 We can't tell when we are stressed and how stressed we are. It's too difficult to figure out.

Truth #10 It is easy to recognize when we are stressed. Using the Stress-Meter, you can check your stress levels.

The ultimate truth is that all stress comes from attachment to thought.

DR. CALM'S PRESCRIPTION

1 ✓ Whatever you believe deeply in your heart is going to determine your destiny. As you believe, you act, and as you act, you reap the results.

2 ✓ You need to be careful what information you let into your mind lest the information doesn't solidify into deep-rooted beliefs. Once solidified into strong beliefs, it is not easy to break-away from them. Therefore, be ever selective in the ideas you entertain.

3 ✓ Refute wrong ideas and false beliefs. Your unknowing allegiance to false beliefs and myths can be detrimental to your growth, happiness, and success. Seek right sources of knowledge early on.

4 ✓ Practice calmness, which will help you wisely discern the good from the bad. You should be like an ant that is able to pick up only the crystals of sugar that are mixed with a heap of sand.

5 ✓ Some myths are deeply rooted, and we don't even know that we are wrong in believing them. The way to uproot them is by self-inquiry and a sincere search for truth.

6 ✓ The greatest myth about stress, deeply rooted in our society, is that "Stress is inevitable, and you have to live with it and there is no escape." Truth be told, *most stress in your life is unnecessary and preventable*. You just need to follow the right teachings.

7 ✓ The ultimate truth is that *all psychological stress is an illusion created through your own thoughts*. The moment you realize that, all your stress disappears into nothingness.

CHAPTER 6

The Big Bang Theory of Stress

In the same way that you can't defeat an invisible enemy, you can't defeat stress until you unmask its true source.

We talk so much about stress. But what, exactly, is *stress*? Have you ever wondered where it comes from? What triggers it? What happens in your brain and body when you are stressed? What's the mechanism of stress? Are hormones the cause of stress or the result of stress? Is stress a feeling or a symptom? To understand what stress truly is, we need to look deeper. We need to break away from traditional thinking and approach stress in a novel fashion.

Most people equate stress to the signs and symptoms they experience, but are unaware of their state of mind that actually triggered those symptoms

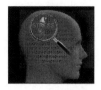 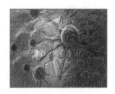 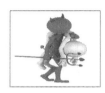

| A Stressed State of Mind | The Release of Stress Hormones | The Signs and Symptoms of Stress |

Figure 6.1. The Three Stages of Stress

What Really Is Stress?

Stress at its core is nothing but a state of mind where you feel unhappy and miserable. And this state of mind results from attachment to thought. Everything else is after the fact. There are three stages of stress (see Figure 6.1).

The Three Stages of Stress

The first and foremost determinant of your stress response is your state of mind. If you perceive a situation to be a threat to you, this state of mind sends signals to your brain to initiate the *second stage*, a stress response by secreting certain substances called *neurotransmitters,** which in turn stimulate various glands in your body to release stress hormones. Your body responds to these hormones in the *third stage*, which leads to signs and symptoms of stress, like anxiety, rapid heartbeat, rapid breathing, sweating, and

---

* A neurotransmitter is a chemical substance that is released at the end of a nerve fiber by the arrival of a nerve impulse and, by diffusing across the synapse or junction, causes the transfer of the impulse to another nerve fiber, a muscle fiber, or some other structure.

so on. Sometimes, the signs and symptoms of stress are subtle with no obvious physical symptoms, but you feel *emotional* distress.

If we look at the cascade of events described above, it is obvious that the *stress response and its adverse effects are a result of your state of mind when you perceive a threat.* Ultimately, this means it is your state of mind that determines whether you become stressed. If you learn to be calm even in the face of a threat, whether real or perceived, that will give you supreme control to deal with the situation. *You literally can bypass the reactive stress pathways in your brain and choose your response proactively.* In that calm state of mind, you become invincible. You gain such clarity and focus in your life that you can leap into the future with great confidence and create the destiny of your dreams.

> If you learn to be calm even in the face of a threat, whether real or perceived, that will give you supreme control to deal with the situation.

You probably have met people who remain calm even in the face of major challenges. They seem very resistant to stress, always joyful, playful, and peaceful. They exude love and kindness. You feel positive and assured in their presence. You have that ability inside of you, too; it's just waiting for you to tap into it.

You Can Swiftly Shift Your State of Mind

From the following example from my life, it is clear that our state of mind determines our outlook toward life and our reactions to external circumstances. State of mind is the beginning point of stress. Your body's stress symptoms are the end point of stress. *If you learn to control the beginning point of stress, you automatically control the end result.* That means if you can choose your state of mind, you can avoid stress and its harmful effects!

Once, my wife and I challenged ourselves to an adventure. We wanted to drive all the way up to the top of Mount Washington in New Hampshire, the highest peak in the northeastern United States at 6,288 ft (1,917 m) and the most prominent mountain east of the Mississippi River. As we drove up the mountain, the road took us through a sinuous pathway, and the trees were in beautiful fall colors. At every turn, new vistas opened up revealing beautiful lakes and mountain peaks. However, the roads were very narrow, and at some places there was just enough space for one car to pass through with no railing or barricade on either side of the road.

I was adventurous and excited. My wife, sitting next to me, initially enjoyed the drive, but as we drove up higher and higher, she became anxious, thinking about the possibility of our car rolling down the cliff even with a tiny mishap. Eventually, she started screaming, becoming sweaty and nauseous. I stopped the car for a moment, calmed her, and continued driving until we safely reached the peak of the mountain. We had a great time at the top of the mountain, enjoyed the scenic views, took terrific pictures, and after a few hours, we got back into the car and started our descent.

Before we started driving down, I explained to my wife the power of our state of mind and how it influences our reactions to external stimuli. It seems that little discussion worked on my wife like a tonic. She shifted her state of mind to a more positive one and regained her calm. Now, on the way down, my wife went to the other extreme. She stood up in the car, and through the open roof, started dancing and taking beautiful pictures and videos as I was driving through the same treacherous road winding down the hill. My heart started beating rapidly. I was concerned that she was too excited. I was completely dumbfounded how she had transformed her state of mind, and as a result, she started enjoying the drive instead of thinking about all the possible bad things that could happen. Finally, we reached the base of the mountain and drove back home with a great sense of accomplishment, excitement, and wonderful memories.

Do Stressors Really Cause Stress?

Now we understand that stress is nothing but a state of mind, the next question to ask is, "What triggers a stressed state of mind? Do stressors really cause stress?" Here is the trillion-dollar answer that melts away all stress.

The concept of stressors, external situations, causing stress is a misnomer. All psychological stress is created finally through an internal mechanism mediated by our thoughts. Your thoughts about the situation cause stress, not the situation itself. See the explanation and Figure 6.2.

Internal vs. External Stressors

Traditional thinking is that something external must happen for us to become stressed. But the truth is, all stress originates from within. Even though an external stressor like loss of a job, illness, divorce, or other challenging life situations can trigger stress, often, even in the absence of any external event, people feel stressed. It is because of an internal stimulus or thought process that triggers stress. Let's take a closer look at this phenomenon.

Have you ever felt stressed when there was nothing bad going

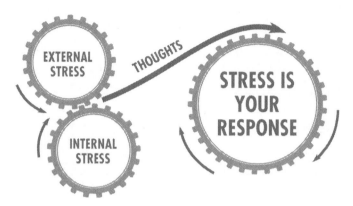

Figure 6.2. Stressors and their Common Link to Stress

on in your life at that moment? I have, and I have tons of examples of people reporting that sometimes they feel bored, unhappy, and miserable for no reason. Then where is the stress coming from? It's not being incited by an external event. Right? In this situation, stress is being generated internally. Sometimes, constant thinking about a past traumatic event or worrying about your future generates stress. These events are no longer present. They happened long back, or they haven't happened yet. But your mind generates stress from within, thinking about these *virtual, unreal events*. I call them *internal stressors*.

All Stress is Generated Within

So, the indisputable truth is, beyond the labels of "external" and "internal," *the final pathway to mental stress is through your own thoughts. So, there are not really any stressors outside of you— all psychological stress originates from within.*

For example, if you are getting divorced, you might keep thinking about certain set of thoughts associated with divorce and stress yourself. The same could be said about a medical procedure that you have coming up; there are certain thoughts associated with it, and you could keep thinking about them to the point where your anxiety puts you in a state of panic. The truth is, it is not the situation itself but your thoughts about the situation that are causing anxiety and worry. I am not saying that you should not think about these problems and not take care of them. You should. What I *am* saying is that most people get caught up in their

> There are not really any stressors outside of you — all psychological stress originates from within.

thinking so much that they get mentally paralyzed but find no solutions. *It is not the divorce, the medical procedure, or some other external event but your persistent thinking about those situations that is ultimately triggering and perpetuating your mental stress.*

This truth is illustrated in the following real-life story.

On Friday evening of a long weekend, you and your friend decided to go shopping. Halfway to the mall, while still on the highway, traffic became congested. As you crane your neck out of the window, you see that there was a terrible accident where a Jeep was overturned at the notoriously steep Exit 48. It seems that the passengers in the Jeep were badly injured and the site was bloody. The police and paramedics are taking care of the injured passengers.

Your friend, who was seated next to you, saw the blood and felt anxious, sweaty, and nauseous. In the next moment she fainted. You saw the same blood, but you were fine . . . you didn't feel any symptoms. You quickly performed first aid and she woke up. You reassure your friend, offer her some water, and she calms down. You slowly drive away from the incident thinking, What happened to my friend? She was perfectly all right one moment and the next moment she suddenly turned into a nervous nelly. You are puzzled by the whole incident. What triggered this stress reaction? Why didn't you have any stress symptoms while your friend reacted so dramatically?

The answer is, each person reacts differently to the same event. When your friend saw the accident, certain thoughts ran through her mind and triggered a stress response from her. (Her thoughts are determined by her past experiences, her outlook toward life, and her state of mind at that moment). If she had not taken those thoughts seriously and had let go of them, she would not have felt stressful at all. A stress reaction would not have started in the first place. You create stress through your own thoughts. Most stress in life is like that! If you take time to calmly analyze a situation and examine your thoughts, it will be evident that all stress in your life is initiated by your own thoughts, consciously or unconsciously!

You think it is the blood that made your friend nauseous and sweaty? It's not the blood itself that made your friend faint; it is her thoughts and perceptions about blood that are responsible for her feelings and reactions. If it were just the blood or accident that caused these symptoms, then everyone who witnessed it, including the policemen and paramedics, should have fainted. Can you imagine that happening? It would have been a total mess on the interstate!!

The Three Truths About Stressors that Make Them Powerless

In the previous section, we understood the true origin of stress, which is our own thoughts. We saw that thoughts finally mediate stress whether it is coming from external stressors or internal stressors. We also noted that the term external stressor is a misnomer because all psychological stress originates within. In this section, we will shed further light on stressors and render them powerless.

1. What Stresses One Person May Not Stress Another

The following real-life example shows how we all react differently to different stressors in life. What stresses one person may not necessarily stress another.

When I was in college, I had a friend, Mary, who used to get stressed over being punctual. She used to prepare hours before any appointment and leave much earlier from home than she really needed to. She used to get very anxious until she reached her destination. It could be an appointment to go to a doctor, hair salon, movie, or a trip to the city. It did not matter what kind of appointment it was. But, her brother, John, never used to stress about time. He used to say, "It's good to be punctual, but there is no point in getting anxious and to keep checking your watch every minute." It didn't bother John if he was a little late. While both were usually on time for their appointments, John was calm, and Mary was anxious. That's the difference. In this instance, time is a major stressor for Mary but not for John.

But one thing John was always worried about was grades. It didn't matter how well he prepared for an exam or how well he performed on it, he always worried about his grades. He would stress himself and everyone around him. But his sister Mary was quite the opposite when it came to grades. She never stressed about grades. She used to say, "What's the point worrying about grades? You do your best on the exam and forget about it. If you worry, it's not going to change your grades." In the end, both usually passed their exams and got good grades, but the difference was, again, one approached this with a cool composure (this time, Mary) and the other with a lot of worry (John). You see here that grades are a major stressor for John but not for Mary.

2. Your Reactions to Stressors Change over Time

Both Mary and John did change over time. Mary does not stress about time anymore nor does John stress about grades. However, one of the things Mary constantly worries about now is her weight. Even though she is neither obese nor overweight, she is meticulously careful about what she eats and what she doesn't to the point where she obsesses so much about her weight that it's impossible for her to enjoy a good meal. However, because of a major health problem she developed, she was finally forced to change her eating habits.

The primary thing John worries about now is money. Because of his obsession to make more and more money, he works nonstop. Most people would consider him financially successful at this juncture in his life, but that does not deter him from devoting his entire time to just making more money, at the expense of his family and health. His life is totally out of balance with little time spent with his wife and children. Eventually, that led to major problems in his marriage. Finally, because of a major relationship crisis, he slowed down and learned the value of a work–life balance. He let go of his strong attachment to money and all the stress that came with it.

3. Your Stressors Themselves Change over Time

What stresses you today may not stress you tomorrow. Do you see how the same people react to different stressors differently at different times in their lives? The point here is, the external event that stresses you today may not stress you tomorrow, and your reaction to the external event changes over time. This is because *you are constantly adapting to your external circumstances.* The fact that you are stressed is not solely because of an external event, even though it may appear so. It is because of an interaction of your mind with the external circumstance, which will lead to either a calm or stressful outcome. *The good news is even though you may not have control over the external event, you have control over how you perceive the event and respond to it.* You have a choice in what you want to do in any given circumstance.

Conclusion: Stressors Are Not the Sole Determinants of Stress

Stressors are not the sole determinants of stress. It is your response to stressors that plays a major role. In almost every situation in life, you have the *choice* whether to get stressed or not. Neither stress nor stressors are constant. They are transient. If you let stressors determine whether you get stressed, then you will always be stressed because this world is imperfect, and you will always face challenges in one form or another. The only way out of stress is to choose your response calmly and wisely in any given situation. *You can allow your thoughts to quiet and calm your mind, regardless of the situation.*

> Neither stress nor stressors are constant. They are transient. If you let stressors determine whether you get stressed, then you will always be stressed because this world is imperfect, and you will always face challenges in one form or another.

DR. CALM'S PRESCRIPTION

1 ✓ Know that the origin of stress is not external. Stress is generated from within.

2 ✓ Be aware of the three stages of stress: a stressed state of mind, release of stress hormones, and manifestation of stress signs and symptoms.

3 ✓ Stress is a state of mind where you feel unhappy and miserable.

4 ✓ A stressed state of mind stimulates a cascade of hormones in your brain and body, thus resulting in the stress symptoms and signs. If you are aware of this, you can eliminate stress at its roots by addressing the state of mind that is causing you distress.

5 ✓ Realize that the terms external stressor and internal stressor are misnomers. Whether it is an external stressor or an internal psychological stressor that bothers you, know both of them affect you through the common pathway: an internal mechanism mediated through your own thoughts.

6 ✓ The fact that different people get stressed for different reasons at different times in their lives proves stressors are not the sole determinants of stress. It is your own response to stressors that determine if you become stressed.

7 ✓ If you find a way to calm your mind and allow the negative thoughts to pass, stressors lose their grip on you.

CHAPTER 7

Rational Brain vs. Impulsive Brain

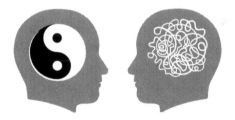

*In the midst of chaos, you feel everything is out of control;
if your mind is calm, you will see order in the chaos.*

I n the previous chapter, we learned that (1) stress is a state of mind and (2) stress originates from within, generated by our thinking. In this chapter, we discover why some people are impulsive and react the way they do, even though they don't necessarily like it. For that, we need to understand the difference between the impulsive and rational parts of our brain.

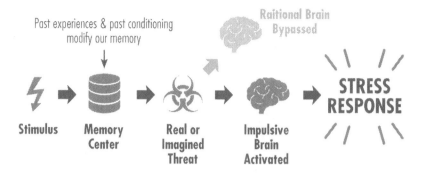

Figure 7.1. Your Impulsive Brain in Action

Why People React the Way They Do

Sometimes, when a threat is imagined but not real, it raises a false alarm. *Your body does not differentiate between a false alarm and a true threat. As soon as the impulsive brain is activated, it initiates a series of actions, beginning with the secretion of stress hormones.* What do you do when you realize that it's a false alarm? Often, people do not know how to turn off the stress alarm or, even worse, they keep setting off their stress alarm inadvertently. This creates a never-ending vicious stress cycle. Is there a way to shut down the stress response and come back to your normal self? Yes, of course. Once you are aware what initiated the stress alarm, you can quickly switch it off and exit the stress cycle.

Your Impulsive Brain Cannot Differentiate Between False and True Threats

Imagine that you are walking on a street in the downtown of a city that you have never visited before. As you walk, you get the feeling that it is an unsafe neighborhood. It's evening, around 6 p.m.; it's just getting dark. It's a new place for you. You suddenly remember that the last time you walked in an unsafe neighborhood you got mugged and robbed. You start getting anxious and sweaty. Your hotel is twenty minutes away. You start walking faster than usual. The next twenty minutes feel like an eternity.

Finally, you reach the hotel. As you enter the lobby, you notice this beautiful young receptionist at the front desk and you approach her slowly, inquiring, "Good evening. How is the neighborhood here? Is it safe at this time of night to walk around?"

She lifts her gaze, looks at you, and answers with a sweet smile, "It's very safe, sir. In fact, this is one of the safest neighborhoods in the whole city. You can safely walk around. Please let us know if you need any assistance from us."

With that answer, you feel relieved. You mumble under your breath, "All the stress I went through was just a waste of energy. Because I felt the environment, the buildings, and the kind of people on the street in this neighborhood were similar to the situation when I was mugged before, I imagined this place to be unsafe. I am glad that it's not."

So, now you walk through the double doors of the main entrance of the hotel out into the night to bravely explore the beautiful downtown neighborhood, enjoying the sights of this new city all around you, and without fear, you walk happily about the streets to reach the restaurant where you wanted to dine that night.

Did you see how your impulsive brain* had imagined a threat based on your past conditioning and experience? Many times, in our lives, even though there is no real threat to us, we still react impulsively because of the influence of past experiences that are deeply engraved in our brains as *subconscious* memories (see Figure 7.1). Our brain is a repository of many subconscious memories and experiences, and they have a strong impact on our present behaviors. But *know that we are not slaves to our subconscious habits or memories. As our awareness levels rise, the unwanted subconscious influences fade.*

The Power of Rational Brain

In the example just presented, instead of impulsively running toward the hotel, you could have called the hotel from your cell phone or you could have gone into the store you were walking by and asked the clerk about the neighborhood. If, indeed, it had been a bad neighborhood, you could have called a cab and waited in the store until the cab arrived or found another way to wisely choose your response. *That's the power of your rational brain.** Your ability to tap into the rational brain and produce creative solutions depends on your ability to quiet your thoughts and remain calm.*

> Your ability to tap into the rational brain depends on your ability to quiet your thoughts and remain calm.

Remember, even when there is a real threat, panic never helps. If you panic, you just run willy-nilly and might even run deeper into danger. When you are confronted by a real threat, your

---

* Impulsive brain is that part of the brain that makes you act on impulse without rationalization. In medical terminology, it's called the limbic system.

** Rational brain is that part of your brain that helps you overcome impulsivity and make rational choices. It's located in frontal lobe of your brain, which is responsible for reasoning, planning, impulse control, problem solving, judgment, and many other higher functions.

hormones will do their job to equip you with the "fight-or-flight response."* If your mind remains calm and clear, you can choose your response wisely and get out of danger.

You Can Bypass Your Impulsive Brain

Here is a good example of a situation during which I bypassed the impulsive brain and used the stress response to my benefit.

> Recently, I visited Dallas, Texas, on a job-related trip. I finished my work around 4:15 p.m. on Wednesday evening. I had to catch a flight back to Hartford, Connecticut, that evening around 7 p.m. It usually takes around thirty minutes to get to the DFW airport from where I was staying. I had enough time. So, I was relaxed, and I walked to the valet to get my car. I handed my ticket to the lady at the counter who told me it would take twenty minutes to get my car. I said okay and waited patiently in the lobby. Twenty minutes passed by and there was no sign of my car. I went back and reminded her. After many reminders and blank reassurances, finally after forty-five minutes, the valet brought my car back to me. By this time, I was getting a little nervous as it was already 5 p.m. By the time I drove out of the garage onto the street, it was 5:10 p.m. I was getting a later start than I had anticipated, and now it

---

* The fight-or-flight response (also called hyperarousal, or the acute stress response) is a physiological reaction that occurs in response to a perceived harmful event, attack, or threat to survival. It was first described by Walter Bradford Cannon. His theory states that animals react to threats with a general discharge of the sympathetic nervous system, preparing the animal for fighting or fleeing. More specifically, the adrenal medulla produces a hormonal cascade that results in the secretion of catecholamines, especially norepinephrine and epinephrine. The hormones estrogen, testosterone, and cortisol, as well as the neurotransmitters dopamine and serotonin, also affect how organisms react to stress.

was rush hour. As expected, the GPS warned me of heavy traffic. I had been hoping to get to the airport by 5:30 p.m., but now it seemed I wasn't going to get there until 6 p.m. I had one hour to spare, and that time might be just enough to catch my flight if I were lucky and nothing else went wrong. It was imperative that I catch this flight because I had to be at work the next day by 8 a.m.

As I started driving through the rush hour traffic, I reminded myself to return the car to the rental company before I caught the shuttle to the airport. As I drove in to return the car, I realized that I was at the wrong destination. The GPS had taken me to the wrong rental car location!

"God! What do I do now? I am already late." I had no time to think or get frustrated or waste any more time. I turned back, fed the GPS the new address, and raced through the traffic, hoping to reach the correct destination this time. It took me ten more precious minutes to reach the right car rental location; I dropped off the car and ran swiftly to the airport shuttle.

Finally, I was at the terminal by 6:15 p.m. I was still hopeful that they would allow me to check my baggage and board the plane. As I entered the line to the kiosk, I noticed that there were two lines and just a few people in front of me in my line. But I did not have time to even wait for an extra minute or I would miss the flight. I immediately asked the airline representative if he could help me bypass the other passengers and go to the front of the line.

He barked, "You shouldn't arrive late." I explained the situation, how the valet took so long, then I was stuck in traffic, and then my GPS took me to the wrong place. He snapped, "So you are blaming it on the traffic; that's what people usually do." I could not believe what I was hearing. I still remember my immediate reaction at that time. I was very angry, my fists tightened, and my teeth clenched.

I remember thinking, "If he is not going to help, that's okay. But misunderstanding my situation and trying to blame me when I have a flight to catch in thirty minutes is ridiculous." My first impulse was to argue with him. But my rational brain warned me not to. I ignored him and asked my fellow passengers if they would let me go ahead of them. Most of them obliged me, but one guy would not.

He said, "I have been waiting here for ten minutes. Why should I let you go ahead of me?" I told him that my flight was leaving in thirty minutes and I was late because of so and so. He replied, "I don't care. If you are late you are late. I am going first." My adrenaline was pumping at 100 miles per second. I could have gotten into an argument with him, but again, my rational brain warned me against it.

I looked around; there was another person at a different kiosk and I urgently ran to him, dragging my heavy luggage and laptop. I explained my story in a minute. He looked at me strangely for an instant, and I didn't think he'd let me go in front of him, but I was pleasantly surprised—actually, astonished!—when he graciously stopped checking in and let me go first. I do not know his name or who he is, but I am still deeply thankful to him for his help.

The representative at the ticket counter, watching all these strange occurrences, understood by now that I was not going to give up easily without her doing her best to get me on my scheduled flight. She told me my chances were slim to get me on the flight, but she would try her best. The computer she was working on gave her trouble.

Murphy's law at work! A few minutes passed by before she decided to grab another computer. Every passing minute felt like an eternity to me. Finally, and miraculously, she checked me in with no guarantee that my luggage would be on the same flight.

I exclaimed, "That's fine! Thanks for your help," and ran toward the security clearance. On the way, I quickly counseled the other airline representative who had not been helpful, "Sir! If you can't help passengers, at least be understanding of their problems and be compassionate," hoping it would change his attitude toward future travelers.

Luckily, there were not many people at the security clearance. I zoomed through there and ran toward the gate where my flight was about to take off. I hurriedly got my flight ticket scanned, and just as they were about to close the airplane doors, I rushed into the cabin, walked to my seat, and collapsed into it, exhaling a huge sigh of relief.

By this time, I had used up all my energy and was utterly exhausted. My clothes were sweaty and my heart was racing. But the stress response was well worth it. The adrenaline rush had been well utilized. I relaxed in my chair and got a beer (usually I don't buy alcoholic beverages on a flight, but I made an exception this time. I really deserved it. I needed to chill out.). After an uneventful flight—thank goodness!—I finally reached my destination. As I disembarked and walked toward the luggage carousal, I was more than happy to find my luggage waiting for me. And that night, as I was walking toward the parking lot to pick up my car, I swore to myself that I would never use a valet service for parking ever again!

Finding Calm Helps You Override Your Impulsive Brain

In the previous real-world example, I could have been taken over by my impulsive brain many times. But *every* time, I kept my cool and let my rational brain overcome my impulsive brain. For a full hour, I experienced a highly charged adrenaline rush, but I did not lose self-control. I used the adrenaline rush to my advantage.

Sometimes, stressful situations are inevitable. But if you find calm you can block the automatic and impulsive stress response. Even under stressful circumstances, you can emerge victorious. *Your heart might be racing, your body might be sweating, your muscles might be aching, but your mind can be calm and clear.* Your inner wisdom and your rational brain will come to your aid— if you remain calm. From this moment on, let's firmly commit to the idea that we all are going to find calm even in the midst of chaos! That's the only way to evade the stress tiger!

> Your heart might be racing, your body might be sweating, your muscles might be aching, but your mind can be calm and clear.

DR. CALM'S PRESCRIPTION

1   Your body does not differentiate between a false alarm and a true threat. As soon as the impulsive brain is activated, it initiates a series of actions that secrete stress hormones.

2   Often, people do not know how to turn off the stress alarm or, even worse, they keep setting off their stress alarm innocently. This creates a never-ending vicious stress cycle. Don't get stuck in the cycle of stress.

3   Once you understand what initiates the stress alarm, you can switch it off and quickly exit the stress cycle.

4   Sometimes, even though there is no real threat, we react impulsively because of the influence of past experiences that are deeply engraved in our brains as subconscious memories. Know that you are not a slave to your impulsive brain. As your awareness levels rise, your impulsivities fade.

5   When you are confronted by a real threat, your hormones will do their job to equip you with the "fight-or-flight response." If your mind remains calm and clear, you can choose your response wisely and get out of danger.

6   If you develop the habit of calmness, you will be able to handle life's challenges with grace. You will be able to override your impulsive brain.

7   You can rationalize your stress response. You can let your body naturally function when there is a real threat and a stress response is needed, but you can also remain cool headed and allow your mind to function calmly.

CHAPTER 8

Acute Stress vs. Chronic Stress

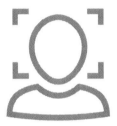

*We cannot recognize what is abnormal
until we realize what is normal.*

How Did Your Ancestors Respond to Stress?

Have you ever wondered how our ancestors responded to stress? Do you ever feel like everyone around you overreacts to stressful situations? Do you feel like some amount of stress is needed to live in this modern society? If so, where do you draw line between the so-called good stress and bad stress? In this

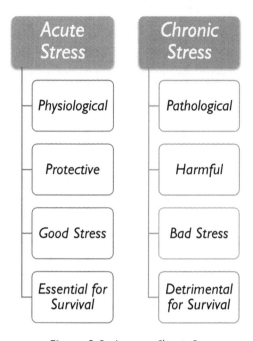

Figure 8.1. Acute vs. Chronic Stress

chapter, we will find answers to these questions and to do that, we need to learn a little bit about the history and purpose of stress in our lives.

The term *stress* was originally borrowed from the field of physics by Dr. Hans Selye in the 1920s to signify an external force causing pressure on a physical body. He noticed that when such external pressure caused strain on the body, patients felt sick. He called it *stress*. But soon other researchers noticed that patients felt stressed even when they experienced psychological events like loss of a job, loss of a loved one, divorce, etc., without any physical pressure on them. That led to the conclusion that stress can be triggered either by physical or psychological events and the response people have to such events is called *the stress response*. So, you may ask, "Is that stress response good or bad for us? Is there a thing called good stress? What's the difference between good stress and bad stress?"

Good Stress vs. Bad Stress (see Figure 8.1)

Yes, there is good stress; if it is an acute stress reaction, which is a normal, protective response to an acutely stressful event like an illness, accident, or a life-threatening situation, that can be viewed as "good stress." This stress response was developed millenniums ago to equip the early humans to deal with the dangers of living in the wild. When early humans faced a wild animal, their bodies needed that alarming stress response—the traditional fight-or-flight response—to provide them with the energy and internal tools to face the threat to life. The rational brain got bypassed, and the impulsive brain took over. *The acute stress response can be considered a good response if utilized well and if you don't lose your rationality while dealing with the stressful situation.*

> The acute stress response can be considered a good response if utilized well.

Physical Threats vs. Psychological Battles

However, in the 21st century, our constant companions changed from wild animals to pet animals and from physical threats to psychological stressors. Most of what you face in this modern world is psychological battles, and it is important for you to handle them gracefully—if you cannot prevent them first. Your body rarely needs the enormous physical power and the alarmingly strong stress responses of the caveman to deal with the challenges of modern day living. *In this modern world, you need different tool sets and skills to survive the tigers of psychological stress lurking in every corner of your mental jungle.*

These psychological stress tigers are far more dangerous and difficult to defeat than the physical threats faced by the early humans. Unfortunately, your body and mind still react the same way as the early humans because of thousands of years of conditioning. You can't completely shut off your stress response system. In fact, you should not do that because you will need it when faced with real threats, however unlikely. But what you can do is to wisely turn it on when there is a real threat and shut off the stress response when it is not needed. You should also learn to recognize false alarms and how to turn them off immediately. This new way of thinking will help you lead a happy, peaceful, and balanced life.

Rationalized Acute Stress Response

When you are faced with a real threat, it is appropriate to have a stress response, but that does not mean you have to be mentally paralyzed with fear or anxiety. You can still rationally choose your response in that situation while your hormones do their part to help. I call this type of response a *Rationalized Acute Stress Response*, during which you remain calm, composed, and purposeful, and choose your actions wisely. This way, you are using your stress response to your advantage. Try it! You will be surprised to see how you can remain calm even in stressful circumstances.

Acute Stress and the Role of Stress Hormones

Most people think that they get stressed because of their hormones. In fact, hormones help you deal with challenges and are not the primary culprit for stress; they are just the messengers— from your brain to your body—sent by your nervous system to relay what your brain is saying. Remember, it is a stressful state of mind that initiates a series of biochemical and hormonal changes in your brain, leading to the so-called stress response.

You might ask, "What about the feeling of impending doom, racing heart, rapid breathing, panic attacks, sweating, and other signs and symptoms that we see in a stressed person?" Those symptoms are the end result of a stressed state of mind, the third and final stage of stress response. We discussed earlier that there

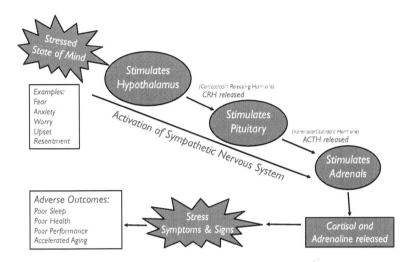

Figure 8.2. The Release of Stress Hormones

are three stages of stress. The first stage is a stressed state of mind, the second is the release of hormones, and the third and final one is the manifestation of stress symptoms and signs (see Figure 8.2).

So, what happens when your stress response is activated? What hormones are released? What do these hormones do to your body, and how do they prepare you for facing the stressful situation?

When you are stressed, your body releases adrenaline, cortisol, and other hormones to help you fight a foe or flee from threatening circumstances. The action of the hormones on your body results in the following (see Figure 8.3):

- Your heart rate increases; your heart pumps more blood into your system to meet the demands of your body.
- Your breathing becomes rapid, and your lungs expand to bring in fresh air and oxygen for your body.
- The blood supply to your muscles increases to allow you to fight or flee.
- Your body quickly mobilizes energy stores into your blood circulation, supplying you with extra energy.

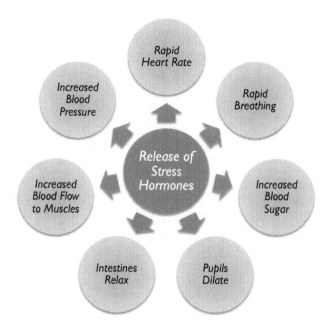

Figure 8.3. Acute Stress Response

All these changes are well organized and executed by your brain and body, supplying you with the tools necessary to face the challenge. It's amazing to see how your body is equipped with very precise mechanisms to handle stressful situations (see Figure 8.1).

Usually, this acute stress response dissipates in 30 to 40 minutes after the stressful event is over. However, the problem with human beings is that we continue to react to the event when it is no longer present, turning it into chronic stress, *the bad stress*.

Do Animals Handle Stress Better than Humans?*

In the wild, once the acute stressful event is over, animals tend to return to their normal state of being. We humans, however,

---

* Animals also go through posttraumatic stress disorder in cases where they were abused. In this example, we are discussing the behavior of the animals under natural circumstances.

often turn an acute event into chronic stress by misuse of our thinking.

Why Zebras Don't Get Ulcers, a book by Dr. Robert Sopolsky, reveals fascinating truths about stress. Though animals react to an acute stressful event with a fight-or-flight mechanism, they don't cling to the stressful event forever like humans do. *Humans tend to misuse their power of thinking and turn that stressful event into a part of their lives and reap chronic stress as a result.*

For example, imagine a lion in the African savannah is hunting down a zebra. If that zebra safely escapes from the lion, after thirty minutes or so, it comes back to its normal state of being. After the acute stressful event is over, the zebra stops reacting to it. It moves on, mixes with the herd, and continues to graze around.

However, let us say you went on an African safari. By accident, you strayed from your group and encountered a lion in the middle of nowhere. You feel anxious and fearful, out of your mind in panic at being stranded and in the grip of danger. The lion walks back and forth for a couple of minutes, considering whether to attack. Suddenly, the lion lunges at you. You try to run away but feel frozen in shock and can't move one inch from where you are standing. Gripped by fear, you close your eyes tightly, expecting any moment to be taken down by the hungry lion.

Suddenly, out of nowhere, you hear a loud bang from a gunshot. The lion, distracted and scared by the noise, stops short of attacking you. Soon, you see the rescue team tackling the lion, which will prevent any further attacks and safely remove you from danger. With a sigh of relief, you run as fast as you can to the safety of the nearest tourist vehicle and slump down in the seat. Feeling exhausted and completely consumed by this life-threatening experience, you are dumbstruck and stay that way for a long time.

Even though your mouth remains shut, your mind does not. For the rest of the afternoon, thoughts run rampant in your mind. You keep rewinding this terrible experience in your mind. You keep thinking about how the lion attacked you in vivid detail. You reach your hotel room and crash on the bed. That night, you are suddenly woken by a terrible nightmare in which you dreamed that the lion has broken your leg and is dragging you down to his den. Waking up in a cold sweat, you realize it's just a nightmare.

The next day, you wake up late but feel tired because you slept poorly. Now, you keep thinking about this experience again and again, and your mind just can't let it go. You tell your story to everyone around the breakfast table and then in the tourist bus. Later, you call your friends who are thousands of miles away and repeat your story. You get empathy and sympathy from your friends and family. You abruptly stop your tour of Africa and return to your home country prematurely. Although the lion has long forgotten you, you haven't forgotten the lion. Even after a week (and sometimes months to years), your mind keeps dwelling on the lion. You fearfully dream of the lion every night and wake up screaming in the middle of the night. In medical terms, this is called posttraumatic stress disorder. Believe it or not, most people experience a milder form of post-traumatic stress disorder at some point in their lives whether they are aware of it or not. Sometimes it is very subtle, and sometimes the symptoms and signs are obvious.

Chronic Stress is a Dysfunctional, Repetitive-Thinking Program in Your Mind

Did you see how a human acts differently than an animal facing a similar threat? The event shakes you up so much that you think about the lion day and night! "Why is this lion attacking me? There are 100 other people who came along with me to this safari. Why not them? Why am I alone involved in this? I am a good person. I never caused any harm to this lion. I am an animal lover. I even have three cats and four dogs at home, and I take care of them very well. This lion should be informed about my good nature. I can't believe this lion attacked me." And you keep on repeating this illogical thinking, then tell this horrible experience to everyone around you. You make this story a part of your life (while the lion has long forgotten you, you haven't). *Human beings misuse their thinking and create chronic stress in their lives.*

Stop Pressing Your Own Buttons — Don't Get Stuck

Remember, to the degree we get attached to past stressful events, to that degree we suffer from chronic psychological stress. When bad things happen in life, we cling on to them much harder than animals do. We, as humans, tend to turn an acute stressful event into chronic stress by misuse of our thinking. *If we stop misusing our thinking, we will find the serenity and peace in our lives.*

Did you ever notice what happens to a CD that is stuck while spinning? It keeps repeating the same song again and again. Likewise, sometimes you endlessly repeat the same thoughts again and again in your mind. Because of this, unfortunately and often unconsciously, you get into a negative or stressed state of mind and create unhappiness for yourself and the people around you, often your loved ones. You basically

> If we stop misusing our thinking, we will find the serenity and peace in our lives.

get attached to a thought and make it your reality. Often, the reality created in such a negative state of mind is miserable. Why create such an unhappy reality for yourself? The following real-life example demonstrates this point well.

A few years ago, one of my friends became interested in the stock market when it was at its peak. He listened to his stockbroker's advice and started investing large sums of money. He became excited as soon as he made some profits. He did well for a few weeks, and then suddenly the market crashed and the stock value plummeted. He panicked and started selling his stock and lost a lot of money. He went through so much stress at the time that he had a mental breakdown.

He was worried about all the money he lost and what would happen to his future. He kept thinking and telling himself that he should have never listened to the broker's advice to invest in the stock market! He could not sleep well. He kept thinking that if he had only kept his money in a savings account at least it would have grown by the 0.5 percent interest offered by his local bank! He had intended to use that money to buy a house next year. Now what was he going to do? He felt that his future looked horrible! He did not see a way out of the problem. This self-criticism, negative thinking, and constant worry went on for a while.

He swore that day that he was never going to invest his money in the stock market again. His family and friends consoled him. Even though he is an intelligent man and started taking corrective actions, his thoughts of self-criticism were eating him up inside. At last, after three months, he finally came out of this stressful spell and started feeling better. All this time, he had refrained from calling the stock broker or responding to the broker's calls. Now, deciding to take out whatever money he still had left in the stock market, he calls the broker.

The broker answered, "Almost two months ago, I called you many times, but since you were angry with me you did not answer my phone calls. At that time, suddenly, the market recovered for a short period of time, and I was able to recover most of your investment. If you had not been angry with me and answered the phone, you would have made some profits, and more importantly, saved yourself all this heartache!"

This news was completely unexpected, and my friend was happy that he came out of the situation unscathed. He regretted being angry at the broker, but he stuck to his decision that he was never going to put his money in the stock market again.

In this example, my friend got stuck in his thinking. It is understandable that he had every right to be unhappy about the money he lost, but *the real problem was he could not stop thinking* about it. He dug himself into a deep pit of misery, self-pity, and self-blame. Moreover, he started imagining a fearful future. Regardless of what kind of thoughts you have (whether they are about the past or the future), if you get attached to those thoughts, they inevitably cause stress. In that poor state of mind, you can't see solutions to your problems.

In the end, my friend realized that *he magnified his suffering by misusing the power of thought*, that is, by his inability to let go of the negative thoughts in his mind. If he had realized the truth that *no matter how dire a situation looks now, if you learn to remain calm and avoid being trapped in a negative state of mind, the solution will always appear,* he would have saved himself from a lot of stress.

Chronic stress is never good. It's harmful. When your body is taxed with chronic stress, your ability to respond to acute stressful events becomes more challenging. A chronically stressed person when faced with a major stressful event may have a sudden increase in blood pressure and heart rate that can trigger a heart attack or stroke or other devastating health problems. That's the reason why *you should not let even an inch of chronic stress creep into your life.*

DR. CALM'S PRESCRIPTION

1 Recognize that an acute stress response is a normal physiological, protective response to an acute life- threatening event. Its purpose is to prepare you to face the threat or escape it. It is "good stress."

2 Acute stress should dissipate in 30 minutes or so in the absence of continuing threats. Anything beyond that, you need to examine why you are feeling constantly stressed.

3 Chronic stress is pathological. When you continue to respond to a stressful event that is no longer present, you create chronic stress. That is *bad stress*. Avoid chronic stress by all means.

4 Most chronic stress is self-inflicted. It results from an unhealthy, obsessive repetition of your thoughts. Basically, as human beings, we run a dysfunctional, repetitive thinking program in our minds that leads to chronic stress.

5 Don't keep reacting to an event of the past or imagine a fearful future, lest you inflict unnecessary stress on yourself.

6 Unlike animals, humans misuse their thinking and magnify their suffering. Put a brake on your restless thinking and eliminate chronic stress from your life.

7 In modern society, we mostly wage psychological battles, not physical ones. Finding calm in the midst of chaos is the quintessential skill to surviving 21st-century stress. Master that skill.

CHAPTER 9

How Full Is Your Stress Pot?

Don't let stress accumulate in your life. Stress begets stress.

Why Do People Overreact?

Did you ever wonder why people overreact to little things? Why do good people do bad things? Why do people get depressed over seemingly minor problems? Why do people commit suicide? What makes a person take his or her own life? For people to take their own life, something must be terribly wrong in their personal world. How do they get to that point?

These are deep and serious questions. And understanding the relationship between resilience, innate health, and chronic stress enables you to be compassionate with these individuals and help them instead of judging or labeling them.

Chronic Stress Reduces Stress Threshold

Chronic stress accumulated over a period is called *allostatic load* or *chronic stress load*. *Allostatic load* is harmful to your health; it reduces your "stress threshold."* If you are suffering from chronic stress, you might get irritated easily and every little thing bothers you. The following example demonstrates that.

It is Thursday evening, and you are almost finished with your work week. You feel relaxed, and you are upbeat as you arrive home. You pull your car into the driveway, open the garage door, and even as you are parking your car, you hear a happy and familiar voice approaching you with such joy—your six-year-old daughter is excited to see her dad come home from work so early that day. You reach out to her with excitement, too! You hug her, kiss her, and go inside together. You take out her favorite ice cream and hand it to her. Then you have a great evening together with the rest of the family and go to sleep feeling fulfilled.

The next day, you wake up and go to work early, intending to have a shorter workday so that you can go out for a movie with your family. However, your workday turns out different than what you expected. You have a long,

---

* Stress threshold is your threshold to get stressed. If your stress threshold is high, you will not be stressed easily, even with major challenges in life. If your stress threshold is low, you will get stressed easily even for minor problems.

exhausting, and stressful Friday. So, you come home late, and as you park your car, your six-year-old daughter jumps on you, expecting you to be nice just as you were the day before. But being tired and stressed, you snap at her, and she is completely taken aback by your angry outburst. She gets startled by your reaction. She does not understand why the same behavior that had won her many kisses and hugs the day before now elicits this unpleasant reaction. She goes away unhappily.

Can you imagine how confused your daughter will be? She does not comprehend what makes you happy and what makes you unhappy. If this happens a few more times, she might withdraw from you completely and just mind her own business without getting too close to you. Do you see what stress can do to you? It can make you look like a monster to others who are affected by your stressed behavior. You may have your rightful reasons to be stressed and behave badly, but people don't often see it like you do. Stressed behaviors lead to stressed relationships, whether it is with your family, friends, or colleagues. As stress accumulates, it causes not only emotional and behavioral problems but also serious physical health problems. Therefore, keep stress at bay.

The Ultimate Disconnect — Lost Soul Syndrome

People often get caught up in a chronic, vicious cycle of stress. The final consequence of relentless stress is a lost soul at the doorstep of failure, disconnected from nature, one's self, and the Higher Power. I call it *the lost soul syndrome*. If you identify yourself or someone else as having some of these characteristics listed, please immediately find help without wasting time!

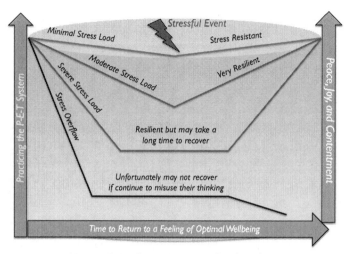

Figure 9.1. Chronic Stress Load and Resilience

1. Forgetfulness and misidentification of your true self
2. Confusion within and without
3. Disconnected from nature, self, and the Higher Power
4. Loss of focus and purpose in life
5. Misuse of your power and potential
6. Loss of hope and feelings of despair
7. Relationships look futile
8. Money and possessions make no sense
9. Anger and frustration about everything
10. Severe depression and thoughts of suicide

The Relationship Between Chronic Stress, Resilience, and Mental Well-being

We can classify people into four types based on their chronic stress load, resilience, and mental well-being (see Figure 9.1). See which category you can relate to:

1. The first group represents people who are stress resistant. They have a minimal stress load in their lives. They have a

good understanding of the P-E-T system or similar teachings. When something bad happens in their lives, they are very resilient and bounce back to a peaceful state of mind immediately. They don't let stress accumulate in their lives by keeping their stress levels low consistently. We can easily recognize such people around us. They are always cheerful, friendly, kind, and compassionate. It's hard to ruffle their feathers! Our aim is to develop such unshakable peace of mind.

2. The second group represents people who have already a moderate amount of stress load accumulated in their lives. Most people fall into this category. When a bad event occurs, they get stressed. They stay in that stressful state for a period but fall back to a peaceful state of mind eventually.

3. The third group represents people who have already accumulated a lot of stress in their lives. Because their stress loads are high, they are deeply unhappy. When something bad happens, they have extreme difficulty overcoming negative emotions. It takes a prolonged period before they can regain their normal state of mind and be happy again. These people need lots of support, understanding, and love to recover. They might exhibit negative behavior such as periodical outbursts of anger or upset feelings. It is not always easy to be compassionate toward them especially if we just look superficially at their bad behavior. However, if we realize that they are behaving badly because of their chronic stress load and unable to handle stress, it will allow us to be more compassionate towards them. The number of people falling in this category has been increasing because of the tremendous levels of pressures we face in the modern world.

4. The fourth and final group represents those unfortunate people who have their lives filled with stress to the brim,

and any shaky event in their lives poses grave danger. Their stress load is so high that when a bad event occurs, they cannot deal with it at all. They are severely depressed and prone to injure themselves or others and possibly commit suicide. Looking from the outside, we might think, "Oh, come on! There is no need to commit suicide over this little issue." But these unfortunate people have accumulated so much stress in their lives that even a minor event can tip the scales to the other side. If our health care practitioners pay attention to the chronic stress levels in their patients' lives and its relationship to depression and suicide, they could help these people heal much faster rather than simply pre-scribing medications alone to treat them. Unconditional love, understanding, compassion, not judging or labeling them, and expressing belief in them helps their mental health to be restored and goes a long way in healing them.

Regardless of how you categorize yourself, how long you have been stressed, and how much stress load you have accumulated in your life, the indisputable truth is that you have an innate capacity to be resilient and to reclaim your mental well-being.

Calmness Lights the Fire of Wisdom and Burns Stress Away

As the fire from a single match can burn up mountainous heaps of hay, so, too, the fire of wisdom can quickly burn away all the stress you have carried with you.

With deep conviction born out of multiple life experiences, I can vouch for this truth. Throughout the history of this world, the power of human resilience has triumphed time and again against the odds of life's biggest challenges. So, stay put. Stay strong. Determine and decide today to learn the P-E-T system so that you might *ignite the fire of wisdom in the cave of calmness to burn up the darkness of ignorance,* which is the root cause for all stress.

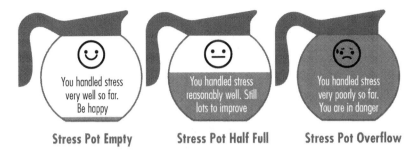

You handled stress very well so far. Be happy

Stress Pot Empty

You handled stress reasonably well. Still lots to improve

Stress Pot Half Full

You handled stress very poorly so far. You are in danger

Stress Pot Overflow

Figure 9.2. Measure Your Stress Pot

The deeper your practice of the P-E-T system, the faster you will recover from stress and reclaim your innate health. And that is what the rest of the book is about.

Check Your Stress Meter

The human mind is a jungle in which the deadly tigers of anger, greed, hatred, worry, fear, jealousy, and many other negative emotions roam every day. To discover the ten deadly tigers of stress and measure your stress levels, visit StressFreeRevolution.com and click on **Check Your Stress Meter** link. This scale measures and warns you about your stress levels, how full your stress pot is, and the action steps to be taken (see Figure 9.2).

To Exit the Stress Cycle, Empty Your Stress Pot Often

Take some time off from work and all routine activities on a regular basis to unwind and give your mind a break from worldly problems. Relax and refresh. When you go on vacation, go with the intention to relax and rejuvenate. Unfortunately, the number of vacation days has been shrinking for most people, and although people go on vacations, they carry their work and family stress right along with them. Cell phones and laptops are making it difficult for people to relax on their vacations. The Internet has become all-pervasive, invading the privacy of even newlywed

couples who are supposed to be on a romantic getaway! Your mind
is not off from work if you constantly check e-mails and important
work-related messages as your partner is patiently and grudgingly
waiting for your undivided attention. When you go on vacation,
be on vacation!

More than ever, *now* is the most important
time to learn how to tame the tiger of stress so
that you can remain refreshed and relaxed not
only during vacations but also in your everyday
life. If you are calm, composed, and happy in
your daily life, then you will carry that with you
when you go on vacation.

> When you go
> on vacation, be
> on vacation!

If you practice the P-E-T System espoused in this book, you
won't have to wait for your vacation to find peace of mind. You
can remain relaxed and peaceful every day of your life! Every
weekend can be a mini-vacation!

DR. CALM'S PRESCRIPTION

1 Every day, the ferocious tigers of negative emotions in the jungle of your mind roam freely. When you learn to tame these tigers, you will be able to rise above suffering.

2 People react badly to little things because there is too much stress going on in their lives. If you understand that, instead of retorting and saying something bad, you could be more compassionate toward them.

3 Chronic stress reduces your stress threshold. The more stressed you are, the more likely you are going to get stressed even over little things. So avoid accumulating stress in life.

4 People get inadvertently caught up in the chronic stress cycle and feel a disconnect from nature, self, and the Higher Power. This eventually leads to total burnout. Avoid this trap and break away from the stress cycle.

5 Make sure you empty your stress pot often. Relax and recharge your body-mind every day.

6 People who are severely stressed and depressed need more of your compassion than your judgment. When you understand the relationship between chronic stress and resilience, you will be able to provide that deep compassion and care they need.

7 Just because you have been stressed for years does not mean that you will never find peace of mind. Your predicament is not years of stress accumulation but the lack of understanding of the right principles that melt away that stress. Years of stress and mountainous loads of suffering can all be dissolved in a moment with the right knowledge and techniques. You can set yourself free!

Discover the Forces that Shape Your Destiny

Part IV Objectives

- Know that no situation is hopeless. There is always light at the end of the tunnel.
- Discover the four forces that propel you out of despair.
- Realize your true nature and tap into your true potential.
- Inner wisdom is the priceless treasure you possess. Make sure you access it.
- Know the limitations of your intellect and complement it with the power of your intuition.

CHAPTER 10

Overcoming Adversity and
Dispelling Despair

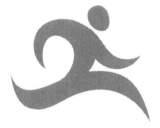

Life is not a sprint; it is a marathon.

No Situation Is Hopeless

There will be times in your life—no matter what you do and how hard you try—when life's challenges will cause extreme misery and sorrow. It is as if all your efforts are in vain. You feel as if you are stuck in a tunnel of despair. Everything around you looks dark and uncertain. It seems like things are falling apart and your world is coming to an end. It's very hard to see a way

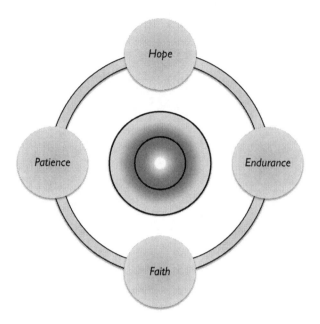

Figure 10.1. The Four Forces that Dispel Dispair

out of your problems when you are stuck in the tunnel of despair. During these times, there are four essential thought forces that can help you overcome adversity and despair (see Figure 10.1).

Hope

First, there is *hope*. Without hope, nothing moves forward in life. People can do terrible things to themselves and others when they feel hopeless. They might commit suicide or even think about killing others. Consequently, the most important thing you have to develop is the power of hope. You should never say your situation is hopeless; to say that your situation is hopeless means that you doubt the infinite power you have within you.

This universe is not designed to be scarce. The default design of this universe is abundance. Our universe is designed to provide for all the needs of the trillions of living beings in this world with abundance. Those who find strength to see at least a ray of hope, even in the darkest hours of their lives, will definitely find a way out of their problems. This is an inescapable truth of life. It is the power of hope that helps people see the light at the end of the tunnel. The stronger the feeling of hope, the easier it is to emerge out of the tunnel of despair.

Faith

But hope alone is not sufficient to emerge out of the tunnel of despair. Although you see the light at the end of the tunnel, you also need to make an effort to emerge from it. As you travel through this dark tunnel of despair, your abilities will be tested and doubt will arise in your mind. The beginning of doubt in your mind means the beginning of the erosion of your self-confidence. But during those times of self-doubt, it is the power of *faith* that propels you forward. Deep inside, if you have faith that things will get better no matter how difficult your situation is today, it will help you overcome your self-doubt. Know that this universe is designed not to fill you with doubt and despair, although for a superficial thinker it might seem so. Life tests and challenges you to ignite your willpower so that you might awaken your innate and infinite abilities to overcome these challenges and move closer to perfection. And with this power of faith, you will move forward swiftly in life.

Patience

As you propel yourself forward through this tunnel of despair, with faith and hope, you still might not find the solutions that you are looking for. Sometimes, it seems as if there is no end to this tunnel. To emerge successfully, along with faith and hope, you also need *patience*. Be patient until you reach the other end of the tunnel where it is full of light, where you see everything clearly and find what you want in life. You just can't say, "I am hopeful and have faith and I need solutions right away. I can't wait!" Well, sometimes you might get your answers immediately but not always. *Patience is a virtue.* Those people who do not have enough patience will lose in their lives despite any other great capabilities they have. So, keep trying and stay patient. If you do so, it is absolutely certain that you will emerge victorious from any difficult and dark situation in your life.

Endurance

As you move forward with patience, your *endurance* will be tested. Obstacles might arise in your path. With every obstacle, make sure that your resolve to succeed gets stronger and not weaker. Life is not a sprint; it is a marathon. To run a sprint, a short burst of energy is sufficient. But to run a marathon, you need to maintain sustained levels of energy and endurance. The only way to develop this endurance is to keep trying and pushing yourself forward tirelessly through all obstacles. One day, you will develop so much endurance that you will finally run the marathon of your life with ease. Although everyone and everything around you is falling apart, you will remain strong and unshakable. Imagine yourself having that invincible power of an absolutely calm state of mind. Such a feeling is very uplifting and will provide you with energy and endurance to move forward despite all obstacles in your path. You finally emerge from the tunnel of despair, penetrating the darkness around you. Bathed in that revealing, brilliant light at the end of the tunnel, you feel relieved, refreshed, and rejuvenated.

> With every obstacle, make sure that your resolve to succeed gets stronger and not weaker.

The following experience from my life demonstrates the power of the four forces.

At one time in my life, I was in deep distress and felt like my life was about to fall apart. There was a major conflict between two of my very close family members and I was caught in the middle. I felt that the emotional pain and suffering during that stage of my life was enormous. Both family members were important to me, and for the well-being of my family, I couldn't see either one of them hurt or unhappy. I tried everything I could, but I could not find a solution to bring them together again. I thought, "What's going on? I am the stress management expert, and I can't even keep my own family happy and stress-free?"

Thoughts of despair, anger, frustration, and fear surrounded me. I felt stuck in my life. I did not see a bright future. It was during those extremely tough times that I discovered these four forces of hope, faith, patience, and endurance, which helped me to successfully and happily emerge from the tunnel of despair and find a win–win solution for all. Remember, sometimes even though you know that you are doing the right thing and you are applying all the right principles, life still has its own timeline and way of sorting things out. Be patient. When the time is right, things will settle down by themselves. Meanwhile, it is important to stick to the right path and not be impulsive and impatient.

During that time, I was feeling very impulsive and I could have easily said nasty things to the others around me, which would have further jeopardized the relationships. "But," I asked myself, "is it the right thing to do? Should I say nasty things impulsively?" The answer from my conscience was very clear. Do not do it! So I didn't, and I am glad that I didn't. After enduring the situation for many months, with continuous, open communication, affirming the love and affection that I have toward each of my family members, I was able to connect everyone together again. Everyone was happy. Everyone learned from their mistakes, all the negative energy dissipated, and positive feelings were restored.

Remember, there is always light at the end of the tunnel. As you get closer and closer to that end, the presence of that light will be more and more evident. Just make the effort to go all the way through the tunnel!

DR. CALM'S PRESCRIPTION

1   The most important thing we all must develop is the power of *hope*. We should never say our situation is hopeless.

2   Know that this universe is not designed to be scarce. The default design of this universe is abundance.

3   The stronger the hope, the easier it is to emerge from the tunnel of despair. So, always keep your hopes high, even during the severest of trials you face.

4   The beginning of doubt in your mind means the beginning of erosion of your self-confidence. But during those times of self-doubt, it is the power of *faith* that propels you forward. Strengthen the power of faith within.

5   To successfully emerge from difficult situations of life, along with faith and hope, you also need *patience*. It is certain that you will emerge victorious from any dark situation in your life if you practice patience.

6   With every obstacle in your path to success, make sure that your resolve to succeed gets stronger and not weaker. That is a prerequisite for victory in life.

7   Life is not a sprint; it is a marathon. To run a marathon, you need to maintain sustained levels of energy and develop *endurance*. With increasing endurance, life becomes easier.

CHAPTER 11

Finding Guidance during
Times of Uncertainty

*You can rely on your inner wisdom to guide
you out of the maze of life's problems.*

Life Is a Maze with Many Surprises

Life is a complex maze with thousands of convolutions and millions of surprises. You never know what problem is hidden in the dark corners of uncertainty. Life has a knack of startling you when you least expect it. Some surprises are good, whereas others are not. When everything is going fine, suddenly a crisis

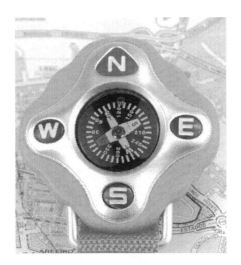

Figure 11.1. Inner Wisdom – Your GPS

erupts like a volcano from the seemingly peaceful ocean of life. Many times, my nerves were tested and stretched to the limits, and my ability to remain calm and centered was challenged.

Don't you wish that you had the ability to predict future challenges in your life with certainty so that you could be better prepared to face them? Unfortunately, none of us have a crystal ball. Maybe you don't want to know every detail about your future, but you certainly need a tool that can prepare you to confidently face whatever challenges may arise, so you can safely emerge from the maze of problems.

Once, my cousin and I decided to visit a mutual friend. I was sitting relaxed in the passenger seat, and my cousin was driving the car. He input the address on the GPS, and off we went. After driving for half an hour, we were still on the road, trying to find the location. We called our friend and he confirmed that we had the right address. We again confirmed the address in the GPS and drove around. The GPS was telling us that we had arrived at the destination, but we could not find the exact place we were looking for.

I thought, "Something is wrong. It can't be this difficult to find this place." I asked my cousin what GPS he was using. He showed me the GPS app on his phone. I exclaimed, "Ah! That's the reason. The GPS you are using is dysfunctional and the maps are not accurate." I opened another GPS app on my phone, and in less than five minutes, we were at our destination.

Do you see how using the right guidance system was so important in reaching your destination in a timely manner?

Similarly, tapping into your calmness-born, intuitive wisdom is pivotal to reach your destination in life successfully. Inner wisdom is your GPS (see Figure 11.1) that helps you navigate the maze of life. Unfortunately, for many people, that inner GPS is dysfunctional due to their restlessness.

Your Inner Wisdom Has the Solutions to All Problems

Each time you calm down, an invisible, inner guiding force comes forth and shows you the solution to your problems.

The following example from my life illustrates this truth.

It's the end of September; already, there's a slight chill in the air in Hartford, Connecticut. I have been waiting for this day for a long time. After much planning and organizing, I am about to fly to the west coast for a much-awaited stress management project. Inwardly, I was feeling very lucky that I had found a very talented team to work with me. On one hand, I was very excited, but on the other hand, I was quite concerned, too. The reason for my concern was because I had not had enough time to prepare for my presentation.

I had set aside a good amount of time to prepare for this project. I had intended to be well prepared, but ever since I had scheduled it, I barely had found enough time to create the necessary material for this project to take off. I had spent a significant amount of money on the consulting company that was going to shoot the videos, and it was very important that this opportunity went well.

For six weeks, as much as I tried, I had not taken a single day off from work because we had had a very busy schedule at the hospital and there was additional pressure to see more and more patients each day. My director had to pull me into work every single day of all the six weeks before this project. As the deadline was getting closer, I started feeling very uneasy. Finally, I told my boss that I needed three days off before my scheduled date of the video shoot so that I could prepare for this project. Graciously, he arranged the time off for me at my request, but an unexpected problem came up that consumed my time on those three days. I had to travel for an urgent meeting out of state, and my valuable time was entirely consumed. I finished that meeting and came back home, and I barely had time to prepare the script.

The problems did not end there. On the day I was to fly to Los Angeles to work on this project, I was supposed to go to the hospital first, finish work, and then drive to the airport to catch a flight around 3 p.m. My schedule was tight that morning. Knowing that, the night before I diligently packed my luggage, ticketed my flight online, and then went to sleep with a sense of excitement that I was all prepared to fly the next day.

I woke up the next morning expecting to have an easy day before catching my flight. But fate had different plans. On my way to work, a crisis erupted out of nowhere. One of my family members was facing a situation of grave concern. I had to spend the next hour and a half trying to settle this issue. In that process, I was pulled into the vortex of intense emotions, and I felt drained at the end of the conversation. All the excitement about the trip died away. I arrived very late to work and was already behind schedule.

As I was trying to quickly finish my work that morning, around 11:30 a.m., to make my situation even worse, I got a text message from the airlines that my flight to LA that evening had been canceled because of a fire in the airport where I had a connecting flight. What the hell! Why was I facing one problem after another? Where were these obstacles coming from? It seemed that fate was trying to thwart my grand plans for success. But I did not give up. I had learned from my previous life experiences that neither failure nor fate can defeat you as long as you don't give up!

I repeatedly called the airlines, but I could not get in touch with them; all I kept getting was a busy signal. So, I decided to drive to the airport to see if they could accommodate me on a different flight. I quickly finished the last few things I had to do at work and left for the airport.

I drove to the airport, parked my car, and walked toward the airline terminal. To my dismay, the flight attendant at the kiosk was not at all polite, compassionate, or helpful in assisting me to find another flight that evening. I was going to lose a lot of money and a great opportunity if I didn't make it to LA on that flight that evening. And I was upset by the whole series of events that had been going on since the morning. A complex mixture of negative emotions including worry, anxiety, anger, and self-pity inundated me and started taking over my rational brain.

Right at that moment, I caught myself in that bad emotional state and said to myself, "Calm down. There is no point getting worried. Worrying only makes things worse. First, calm down and your inner wisdom will show you a way out of the problem." I reminded myself that, "I am more than my emotions. I am more than the events that surround me. I am more than what's going on in my life at that moment." I took a moment to compose myself, took a few deep breaths, practiced a relaxation exercise for a few minutes, and calmed down.

> I am more than my emotions. I am more than the events that surround me.

Once I calmed down, my inner wisdom kicked in and started suggesting alternative solutions. A brilliant idea struck me like a flash of lightning! My right hand quickly reached for my mobile phone in my pocket. I started searching quickly for all possible flights that evening going to LA. As I scanned through the list of flights ... there you go ... I found a flight going to LA later that evening with a different airline than the one I had for my first reservation. I purchased a ticket that didn't cost that much and flew to LA that night. I felt relaxed and relieved. Another great idea popped up in my mind: contact the previous airline to process a refund for my canceled flight. The next few minutes, I spent talking to the airline, explaining the situation. This time, the customer representative was nice. He gladly refunded my money. Happily, I walked through the security line, cleared it, and went on to board the flight. By the time I arrived in LA, it was late at night but I was glad I made it, even though a little delayed, and my team was immensely relieved to see me. They had been quite concerned about whether I could make it happen and arrive as scheduled—and miraculously, I did!

The Only Certainty during Times of Uncertainty

In this scenario, do you see how life is so uncertain? The evening before, I had been 100 percent certain that I was going to wake up in the morning, have a perfect family situation, a good day at the office, a guaranteed flight, and an easy and relaxed trip to LA. But fate had other plans. All the certainties in my life at that time were suddenly transformed into uncertainties with a flick of the magic wand of fate! But with certainty I can say, *If we learn to be calm and find our inner wisdom, it will always show us a solution and guide us out of the maze of problems* (see Figure 11.2). Time and again, this truth was proved to me through a variety of life circumstances. *Your inner wisdom never fails.* All you have to do is to calm down and allow your inner wisdom to surface.

Finally, *life is so uncertain that we don't know what is going to happen tomorrow to our loved ones, our jobs, to all the money and material possessions we have accumulated. So, enjoy every moment of your life today.* Be kind to your friends, family, colleagues, neighbors, and even strangers. Make the best of what you have today. Cherish every moment in life.

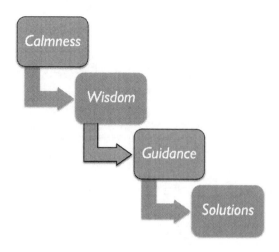

Figure 11.2. Your Internal Guidance System

Treasure Beyond Measure—Your Inner Wisdom

Once, there was a beggar. He sat on an old trunk and begged all day. One day, a wise man passed by, and as usual, the beggar asked for money.

The wise man looked at the beggar for a minute and inquired, "How many years have you been sitting on this trunk and begging?"

The beggar replied, "As long as I can remember."

The wise man asked, "Did you ever open the trunk?"

The beggar looked confused and said, "No one has ever asked me that question nor have I thought about it. Let me open it and see."

And he opened the trunk and much to his astonishment, he found it full of treasure—gold, diamonds, and pearls. He looked at the wise man to thank him for his advice, but he was long gone.

Look inside to your inner wisdom, the greatest treasure you possess. Once you access that treasure, you can stop looking outside for nickels.

Your true nature is priceless and beautiful, like gold. Even when gold is covered by mud, it is still gold inside. It's not tainted. It's not destroyed. Once the mud is washed away, the gold shines through.

In the same way, your inner wisdom, your true treasure is always there with you, too. Sometimes in your life, it gets smeared and covered by the mud of restless thoughts. As soon as you wash away the mud of restlessness, the gold of inner wisdom brilliantly shines through. Calmness is the cleanser of muddy and restless thoughts! Practice calmness every day.

> As soon as you wash away the mud of restlessness, the gold of inner wisdom brilliantly shines through.

DR. CALM'S PRESCRIPTION

1   Recognize that your inner wisdom is your greatest guide. As your inner wisdom blossoms, you find solutions to the problems in life.

2   Uncertainty is part of life. You will face many uncertain situations throughout your life. During those times, your best friend is your inborn wisdom.

3   Develop the power of intuitive wisdom, and it will save you when your intellect fails you.

4   During times of adversity, the only true treasure you possess is your inner wisdom. It is preserved deep within, untainted by all the restlessness and stressful circumstances around you.

5   The moment you regain your calmness, the inner wisdom will come to your aid regardless of how dire your situation is. Practice calmness!

6   Enjoy every moment of your life. You never know what's going to happen next to you or your family and friends. So cherish every moment.

7   Forgive anyone and everyone who could have hurt you knowingly or unknowingly. Life is short. Do not squander your time, resources, and energy. Use them wisely.

CHAPTER 12

The Unfailing Method of Achieving Success

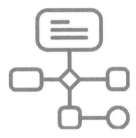

*"What is known is a drop,
and what is unknown is an ocean."*

~ ANONYMOUS

Intellect, Intuition, Insight, and Wisdom

Knowledge is gained in two ways: intellectual learning and intuitive knowing. *Intellect brings information only from the known, whereas intuition brings information from the sources unknown to the intellect.* When you combine both, your chances of

Intellect   *Wisdom*

☐ Powerful but has its limitations	☐ Limitless power and all-knowing
☐ Dangerous and destructive if misused	☐ Always positive and constructive
☐ At risk for analysis-paralysis	☐ Prevents analysis-paralysis
☐ Prone to egotism	☐ Dissolves ego

Figure 12.1. Difference Between Intellect and Wisdom

success are high. In this chapter, we will discuss the definitions of intellect, intuition, insight, and wisdom and their roles in your life.

What is Intellect?

Intellect is the faculty of reasoning and understanding objectively, especially with regard to abstract or academic matters. We discuss more about intellect in the next section.

What Is Intuition?

Intuition is the all-knowing faculty we all possess deep within. When intuition prevails, you know things without the assistance of the information-gathering senses—eyes (vision), ears (hearing), tongue (tasting), nose (smelling), and skin (touch)—and without the intellectual processing of information. Call it gut feeling, the sixth sense, a hunch, or whatever name you want to give it; when you are intuitive, you just know it! And your intuitive faculty works best when your mind is calm and not distracted by restless thoughts. Intuition knows what your intellect knows not.

The following real-life story illustrates how your intuition works. Your intuition works the same way. Turning on intuition is like

Once, I was searching for my phone that had fallen on the floor of my car. It was dark at night, and I had already turned off the car. I was too lazy to start up the car again and turn on the lights. I thought, "It should be easy to find the phone. I know the approximate location of where it fell. All I have to do is just move my hands on the floor of the car and I will find it." I groped in the dark for 5 minutes, but I couldn't find my phone. I was determined to find the phone in the dark, without turning on the lights again. I spent another 10 minutes searching for it and still couldn't find it. With growing frustration, I resigned from that "darkness challenge" and started the car. The moment I turned on the lights, I was able to immediately see the phone sitting in a corner of the car.

turning on a light. When intuition prevails, you see things clearly as if someone shined a light and dispelled the darkness instantaneously. *Calmness is a prerequisite for a well-functioning intuition.*

What Is an Insight?

Insight means seeing from within. When you are calm and intuitive, great insights arise from within. New knowledge dawns upon you effortlessly, as if you have known that knowledge all along. Fresh perspectives flow effortlessly. You don't need to try too hard to learn or express yourself. Understanding is coming from within. If you have ever had such an experience, that means you were having an insightful learning experience. It's a stark contrast from cramming, data gathering, information processing, reasoning, analyzing, or any other intellectual activities. Powerful insights originate from within and, subsequently, you understand things in a new light.

What Is Wisdom?

When your intuition prevails, and you gain insights, that insightful knowledge is manifested as *wisdom*. While you can't measure one's intuition or insights as they are internal phenomena, you can sense how wise a person is, and that is an indirect measure of one's intuition. Whereas insight is the internal expression of intuition, wisdom is the external expression of intuition.

The Problems of this World Can't Be Solved by the Intellect Alone

We live in an intellectually predominant world and for a moment, notice what kind of mess we have created—*the great intellectual turmoil*! We are cutting down trees and mindlessly destroying our environment; underworld intellectuals, like the now-deceased Osama bin Laden, are behind the worst terrorist acts; major nations are fueling terrorism in Syria by supplying money and resources; there are wars across the borders of many countries; there is a huge disparity between the rich and the poor; there is adversity and famine in certain parts of the world where babies are dying of starvation while the affluent nations are battling the epidemic of obesity—the contrasts can't be more striking. America spends more money than any other nation in the world and its health care industry is a disaster! How many more terrible examples do we need before we realize the dangers of being run amok by our mad intellectual faculties? We need wise people running the world, not intellectuals alone! That's the only way to solve our problems and bring peace to this world.

The Intellect Is like Nuclear Power; Use It Carefully

The intellect is a powerful weapon you possess, and it plays a vital role in your prosperity and success. You are blessed if you possess high intellectual capabilities. But if misused, that same powerful weapon can lead to your own self-destruction. It's like nuclear power. If expended well, you can generate electricity, but if wrongly used, the same nuclear power in the form of atom bombs can destroy the whole world.

To avoid such self-destruction, your intellect must be constantly guided in the right direction by your inner wisdom. That guidance within is the most reliable source of "right" living. Intellect, backed up by wisdom, makes you invincible, and even

> Your intellect must be constantly guided in the right direction by your inner wisdom.

the toughest challenges of life must bow before you. You seize the glory of victory from the iron hands of fate! You create your own destiny. History is full of great examples of astute men and women saving themselves and their loved ones from severe trials and emerging victorious. A person is called astute when they combine the power of wisdom with their intellect. That is a necessity in life, lest intellect self-destructs (see Figure 12.1).

The greatest example of the misuse of intellect is Adolf Hitler. Cut off from his inner source of wisdom, but highly intellectual, he went on to relentlessly execute many heinous acts that killed millions of innocent people. Ultimately, his misguided intellect destroyed him like a cancer that consumes its own host.

In stark contrast to this stands Mahatma Gandhi, an intellectual who was an attorney by profession but also an astute man who let his inner wisdom direct his intellectual capabilities to bring the whole nation of India, 300 million people at that time, to one path—the path of freedom and victory—in a nonviolent fashion. That's the power of intellect when combined with the power of wisdom. The reason why

Hitler failed ultimately is because the double-edged sword of intellect turned destructive due to lack of guidance from his inner wisdom.

The Many Merits and Definite Defects of the Intellect

Intellect helps you reason, analyze, plan, deduce, write, understand, and perform many other practical functions. But *the very fundamental limitation of intellect is its dependence on our senses to gather information.* But we know that our senses are limited. Your eyes can only see visible light, the wavelengths of about 390 to 700 nm—called VIBGYOR. Then what about those light particles a human eye cannot perceive? They exist, but we can't see them. The same applies to the perception of sound vibrations. The human ear can only hear frequencies ranging between 20 Hz to 20 kHz. What about other sounds in the atmosphere? Just because you can't hear them, you can't deny their existence. Dogs and cats can hear them!

Why Do Intelligent People Act Stupid Sometimes?

You see, intellect is limited in certain ways because it depends on the senses for its information. *Another limitation of the intellect is that it processes the information based on past experiences, social norms, and our environment.* Its perceptions can be biased and distorted by external factors. That's the reason many intelligent people sometimes get it wrong completely. That's the reason we humans, intellectual beings, at times act very stupid and make terrible mistakes. And there is only one way to solve this problem. That is to take the help of your wisdom. Let it direct your intellect. That is a sure way to succeed in life. The good news is your inner wisdom is available for free, and it's a treasure waiting for you to tap into!

The Secret Power of Einstein

Did you ever wonder why Einstein was regarded as one of the brightest minds of the world? Most people quickly answer that question by saying that Einstein had a very high IQ, which is true. But, along with that, there is a hidden power he possessed that was not noticed by this intellectually dominant world. That hidden power he possessed is the power of intuition. If you read any of his quotes, you will find deep meaning and great wisdom in what he says. That's the reason he remains one of the brightest minds of all time, even though many other notable scientists were born before and after him. He did not solely depend on his intellect but unleashed the power of his intuition to expound profound universe-altering theories. Such is the power of combining your intellect with intuitive wisdom. It will make you soar to the highest levels of success in life.

The End of Egotism

Did you ever look up at the blue sky and wonder what lies beyond it? The sky's vastness is incomprehensible to the human mind! When was the last time you sat outside, relaxing in a chair, and gazed into the dark skies of the night? We are so busy in our lives that we do not have time to enjoy nature and these deep and fascinating mysteries of our universe. As a child, when I beheld the starry sky, I used to wonder, "Where do all those stars come from during the night? Why can't I see them during the day? How many stars are there in this universe?"

Astronomers estimate that the observable universe has more than *one hundred billion* galaxies. Our galaxy (called the Milky Way) is home to around *three hundred billion stars*. Can you imagine how many billions or trillions of stars there are in the entire universe—both seen and unseen? Our physicists say that those stars are much bigger than our Sun. And those stars are much farther away than our Sun. That means they are millions of miles away from us, and yet we can still see them. That means they must be colossal if we can see them from such a vast distance.

We Are Tiny Beings in this Universe

Did you ever wonder how small we are, as human beings, compared to these seemingly endless skies, countless number of stars, and the incomprehensibly vast universe? Did you ever wonder when you sat beside an ocean and watched the waves, "God! How big is this ocean? How many millions of living beings does this ocean hold in its bosom? How little I am as a human being compared to all these infinitely vast entities. I don't even know a zillionth percent of what is actually out there in our universe." When I think about these things, my ego feels so tiny and almost disappears.

What my tiny intellect (in the tiny brain in this tiny body) knows is so minuscule compared to what is out there and what is possible in this universe. "Then, how dare I act every day in my interactions with people as if I have the right answers for everything? How dare I assert and impose my opinions on others so strongly, and how dare I hold onto the little truth I know and expect everyone else around me to follow it? How dare I judge others with the little knowledge I have?" Isn't it foolish to behave this way? When you realize how little you know, your ego will be humbled.

Science Can Only Measure What Is Known

We human beings have come so far in our scientific knowledge and medical sciences, and we are technologically advanced, but we haven't even scratched the surface of the deepest mysteries of life and this universe. And *science can measure only those things that are known to our intellect and are manifested; it can't measure what is unmanifested and unknown to the human intellect.* What is not manifested and not known to the intellect has to be known by intuition.

Why Overthinking Doesn't Help

The intellect brings information only from the known. There is so much information unknown to our intellect. That's the reason overthinking and overanalyzing do not usually help. There are times when you gather all the information possible, analyze it, and wonder why you still haven't gotten answers to your problems. You go into an endless cycle of over-analysis without finding the solution and become frustrated. It's called *analysis paralysis.*

The Paradox of Letting Go

But when you just let go and relax, all of a sudden, the answer to the problem comes forth as if you have known it all along. This happens because *when you become calm, the secret door to inner wisdom opens, and the information you need just appears, shedding light on the problem, showing you the solution.* If you understand this truth, trust it and practice it, time and again your innate wisdom will come to your rescue even when you are in deepest trouble.

This innate wisdom blossoms when you are in a calm state of mind and not only shows you the solutions to your problems but also prevents them in the first place. *When wisdom prevails, you make fewer mistakes and thus prevent the endless complications of wrongdoing.*

Always Listen to Your Gut — It Is Your Second Brain

Do you know how important it is to listen to your gut feelings? Some people call it *intuition*; some call it a *sixth sense*. Practice listening to it. Often, we don't listen to it because our minds are so restless and noisy that the gentle voice of our intuition is often suppressed. But when calmness prevails, this gentle voice of intuition will sound like the roar of a lion in the silent cave of your mind and cannot be suppressed, masked, or mistaken. Behold the power of intuition in the cave of calmness!

The following real-life story underscores the importance of listening to our intuition.

A few years ago, I was actively looking to purchase a house, and after six months, I spotted a beautiful house in one of the best neighborhoods in town. It was my dream house—the most perfect house that I had ever wanted in my life. The previous owners had built it in such a wonderful way that even if I had wanted to, I probably couldn't have improved on the design. The house was full of character, the colors on the walls were uniquely special, and some of the doors had great artistic designs. On top of everything, there was ample sunlight and ventilation. The basement was finished and furnished. And there were many more features that my family and I really loved very much. The previous owners had maintained everything in perfect condition. Obviously, I was in love with this house, and I was fortunate to get a great deal on it. I negotiated the contract and applied for the home mortgage loan. I was assured of getting a loan from the bank.

A few weeks passed and things were moving along well. Four days before the closing date, the banker was giving me all kinds of excuses about how the loan couldn't be processed for some strange reasons. Neither I nor my real estate agent with thirty years of experience could understand the logic behind the banker's argument. We spoke with the manager, the vice-president, and president of the organization. All we got were apologies, excuses, and diplomatic answers, but not the truth. I was very upset for a few days and started looking for other banks from which I could get a loan. But they were charging higher interest rates. To make matters worse, the seller also became upset and very anxious and said he could not wait.

So, I had to let go of this beautiful house of my dreams.

I could have renegotiated with the seller, gotten a loan from another bank, and somehow could have closed the deal. But I did not. I said to myself that maybe the universe for some reason does not want me to buy this house. Something within me told me to hold off on buying this house for now. Because of my past experiences where I had ignored my gut feeling and gotten into trouble, I decided to go with my gut feeling this time and not pursue buying this house, or any house, for the next six months at least.

Guess what happened? Five months later, the organization that I was working for got into a major financial crisis, and my income for that year went down significantly. If I had bought the house, ignoring my gut feeling, I would have been in deep financial trouble. In addition, there was a huge, unexpected shift in my family situation that forced me to move away and relocate to a different part of the country, thousands of miles away. If I had bought the house, I would have been forced to sell it and would have lost a lot of money as a result. Remaining calm proved to be my best asset. It helped me make an intelligent decision, guided by my intuition, that ended up being the best decision for my family.

DR. CALM'S PRESCRIPTION

1 ✓ Intellect is your best friend if you use it wisely. It becomes your worst enemy if you misuse it.

2 ✓ Gandhi and Hitler are two extreme examples of intellectuals. One was well guided by wisdom and the other was completely cut off from his inner wisdom. Decide who you want to be.

3 ✓ What is *known* to the intellect is little. What is unknown to the intellect can be known by intuition. Develop the power of intuition along with your intellectual capabilities.

4 ✓ Over-analysis leads to analysis paralysis because the answer to your problems does not always lie in your intellectual capability to think, reason, and analyze. During those times, resting your mind helps you solve the problem at hand.

5 ✓ Wisdom, insight, and gut feeling are all aspects of the same all-knowing intuition—a power we all possess. Develop the power of intuition and tap into your unlimited potentials.

6 ✓ You develop intuition by developing the habit of calmness. The deeper your calmness, the greater your intuition.

7 ✓ When you learn to combine the power of intellect with the power of intuitive-born wisdom, you become invincible to the lashes of fate and snatch victory from its iron hands.

Exploring The P-E-T System: Your Ultimate Solution for Stress

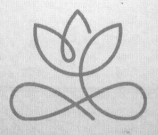

Part V Objectives

- Discover the thief of happiness.
- Understand the Three Principles.
- Learn the relaxation exercises and the calming technique.
- Learn to let go.
- Deepen your calmness.

CHAPTER 13

The Thief of Happiness: Restlessness

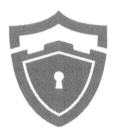

In the palace of peace, the thieves of restless
thoughts steal the crown of happiness, unless
guarded by the soldiers of calmness.

The True Goal of Life

We all want to be happy, secure, and peaceful. There is not a single person in this world who does not want to be happy. Isn't happiness and peace of mind what we all ultimately are looking for in our lives?

Some people might say, "No! Actually, I am looking for money or a great car or beautiful house or some other possession to be attained."

But do you think money or material possessions will give you happiness? Don't we all want money, a house, a car, a good education, and more because we think that these things will give us a sense of security and peace of mind? Money could help us afford a comfortable life, but, money alone can not give you peace of mind.

Professional Success Does Not Necessarily Mean Personal Happiness

If money alone gives us peace and joy, then all doctors, lawyers, business tycoons, and celebrities would be the happiest people in the world. But, as a physician, I can tell you that being a doctor is probably one of the most stressful professions in the world. I have a few attorney friends. They say that their lives are very stressful, too. We see in the news all the time how celebrities are under a great deal of stress; some of them are depressed, some have fallen prey to drugs, and some died by committing suicide. I was shocked when the great comedian and actor Robin Williams committed suicide. What else could anyone ask for in his life? He had fame, money, a great number of fans who admired him, and a lot of material possessions that most people don't have. Do you see how someone could lack happiness and peace of mind even while having a lot of money and material possessions? It is because money and possessions are false sources of happiness. They can only give you pseudo-pleasures.

Your State of Mind Determines Your Happiness

I am not saying that you should forego earning a good salary and live a poor life. Nor I am saying that you should not buy a beautiful house or not go on a great vacation if you can afford those things. But those alone should not be your goals, because those alone will not save you from the misery of the harsh realities of life. You also need to learn how to control your state of mind despite your external circumstances. We all need to practice calmness and unconditional happiness. That's only enhances the joy you derive from the money and possessions you have. *Calmness will make you feel more secure as if you are traveling in a bulletproof car where the bullets of life's toughest challenges will not be able to penetrate the car of your life. Calmness is your protective shield.*

But you might ask, "I always wanted to be calm, but I can't as much as I try. What steals our calmness?"

Restless Thoughts Steal Your Calmness and thus Your Happiness

It is the thieves of restless thoughts that steal the wealth of our peace and happiness. When you are restless, you are automatically stressed and unhappy. When you are unhappy and restless, you make more mistakes. This, in turn, leads to more stress and misery. The vicious cycle continues until you address the root cause of the problem; that is, to dissolve restlessness and reinstate calmness.

Restlessness is like the frost on the windshield of your car—it obstructs your view of the road ahead and prevents you from seeing things in your life with clarity. So, you accidentally run into all kinds of problems. Practicing the P-E-T System will cleanse your mind, dissolve your restless thoughts, and restore calm. It can be as instantaneous as a cleanser cleaning your windshield. *As soon as you become calm, the fogginess of your mind disappears, everything in life becomes clear, and right away you will see the way out of your problems.* In calmness lies happiness and wisdom. A calm state of mind leads to good things in life.

What Causes Restlessness?

But why are most people restless? *Why can't we all be eternally peaceful and joyful?* It is because of our conditioning by society, our

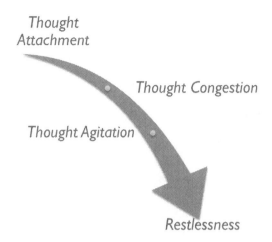

Figure 13.1. The Cause of Restlessness

surroundings, and the people around us. We all are born peaceful and joyful. That's our natural state of mind. Slowly, it gets eroded with time because we are not taught how to use our divine gifts of Mind, Thought, and Consciousness. (see Chapter 14). So, restlessness becomes a habit for us.

The Precursor of Restlessness

Often, restlessness is preceded by thought attachment to a goal or desire. When you set a goal to accomplish or have a desire that is unfulfilled, you get attached to those thoughts. You feel restless until you either accomplish that goal or you accept that you are going to be okay even if you don't achieve it. Only then does your mind rest in peace, at least momentarily, until it is disturbed by another desire, stirring restlessness again. *Thought attachment and thought congestion often precede restlessness* (see Figure 13.1).

No one teaches us these things at home or school. We learn science, mathematics, English, social studies, and more, but not how to be calm. No one teaches us how to face the challenges of life and handle them with grace. *We are forced to learn these things on our own, and life, the greatest teacher, is not always pleasant.* So, we need a science and art that teaches us these skills. That's the purpose of this book. Calmness and even-mindedness are learnable skills, and everyone can learn them.

The Litmus Test for Restlessness

How do we know that we are restless? How do we identify it?

To recognize restlessness: stop whatever you are doing right now. If possible, sit or stand quietly. Watch your thoughts. If they are running in multiple directions, or you are jumping from one thought to another without finishing the previous thought, you are restless. Try to count from one to one hundred without losing the flow of the counting, without losing awareness of what you are doing, without your mind jumping onto something else other than purely counting the numbers. If you can do that, without breaking your flow of thoughts, I think you are in good shape. You are not restless at the moment. But if you are easily distracted and are breaking away from counting, you are restless. The more easily you are distracted from counting, the greater your degree of restlessness.

Restfulness

What is restfulness? How do we define *peace of mind* or a restful state of mind?

Restfulness is the state of a lack of restlessness. In other words, it is a state of mind where you are content with what you have. Your mind is peaceful because your thoughts are restful and not flying in multiple directions, worried about desired outcomes. It is a state of acceptance of things as they are and of what is. It is a state of security that everything was alright in the past, everything is alright now, and everything will be alright in the future, too. It is a state of unshaken faith in yourself and in life.

DR. CALM'S PRESCRIPTION

1 ✓ Realize that the true goal of life is to find permanent shelter in peace and joy. Do not sacrifice your peace of mind for anything.

2 ✓ Know that money and material possessions alone cannot sustain your happiness. True happiness will be ever elusive, unless you learn to control your state of mind.

3 ✓ Thought attachment and thought congestion often precede restlessness and create turmoil in your mind. Do not take negative thoughts seriously and they will go away.

4 ✓ It is your restless thoughts that steal your happiness. Arrest restlessness and reclaim your peace of mind.

5 ✓ Calmness is your protective shield. Learn to remain calm and you will find happiness in life.

6 ✓ Restfulness is a state of acceptance of things as they are and of what is. It is a state of security that everything was alright in the past, everything is alright now, and everything will be alright in the future, too. Be restful.

7 ✓ Contentment is a prerequisite for restfulness. Strive for contentment in life.

CHAPTER 14

The Secret to Calmness: The P-E-T System for Stress-Free Living

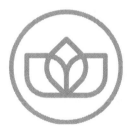

Like you eat food, drink water, and breathe air to keep your body alive and healthy, you practice the P-E-T System to stay calm and keep your mind healthy.

The Discovery of the P-E-T System

Many years ago, when I was in the middle of a perfect storm of stress, destiny had me stumble across certain Principles and techniques that helped me calm down instantly and gave

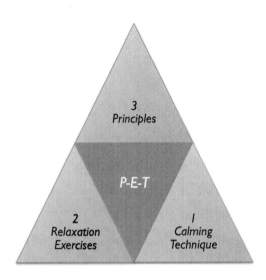

Figure 14.1. The P-E-T System for Stress-Free Living

me the ability to take control of the situation. That ability to calm down in the midst of chaos not only saved my life but also paved a path to the career of my dreams. It was a total transformation of my life.

Over the years, I've faced many hardships and several life-and-death situations. I have put together the lessons I learned and the insights I gained from these experiences into a system called *The P-E-T System of Stress-Free Living*, or P-E-T for short. P-E-T, as represented in Figure 14.1, stands for:

3 **P**rinciples
2 **E**xercises
1 **T**echnique

I recommend you practice this system regularly. It melts away stress instantly and works with predictable accuracy! *A strong determination to be victorious in life, bolstered by the indestructible resilience of the human spirit, can beat all the odds of life's challenges and bestow upon you the gifts of peace, joy, and love.*

The Embattled Soul

Your soul is constantly battling a variety of external and internal forces to keep stress at bay and maintain peace. Many years ago, when I was unaware of these Principles and techniques, I lost this battle quite often, and unfortunately at that time, I did not know why. I thought that being stressed and being unhappy was the norm, with a few touches of happy moments sprinkled here and there. At that time, I did not know it was possible to live life in an entirely different way, where peace, joy, and harmony are the norm, and stress is only a sporadic occurrence.

The Message of Hope

A new world of peace, joy, and harmony opened up to me only after I had my first powerful glimpse into the Three Principles and the calming techniques. As I started practicing these Principles and techniques, my ability to remain calm deepened; the number of victories in my battle between peace and stress started outnumbering the number of defeats. There are times when it seemed that I momentarily lost the battle only to recognize that I could regain my peace of mind immediately. Over time, I realized that *my ability to overcome the challenges and win the tests of life were directly proportional to my ability to remain calm and centered.*

> My ability to overcome the challenges and win the tests of life were directly proportional to my ability to remain calm and centered.

With that knowledge, I developed a new conviction that *we have a fair degree of control in our lives if we practice calmness.* And I believe this is a message of hope for millions who are looking for solace from the relentless march of stress in their lives. If you embrace the P-E-T System and learn how to anchor yourself in calmness, life becomes a journey of success.

You Reap Maximum Benefit by Embracing the P-E-T System as a Whole

Over the course of my life—after many stressful experiences, much study, and practical application—I realized all three components of the P-E-T System are essential for maintaining a calm state of mind, both in the short and long term. Each of these components is unique and promotes peace of mind and happiness in its own way. Tailor the use of the components to your situation and use one or more components as you see fit. In other words, you can mix and match them depending on your situation. You will reap the maximum benefit by practicing all three components daily. In the beginning, you may start with just one component and slowly add the other components into your schedule.

The **P**: The three **P**rinciples are the foundation for human experience. As you come to deeply understand them, all the stress in your life melts away effortlessly. A new joy finds its way into your life. Sometimes, this transformation is almost immediate, and you suddenly break free from all your limiting beliefs and feel elated. Sometimes, the effect is more subtle, less dramatic, and the transformation in your life, albeit slow, is underway. It all depends on the intensity of your desire to sincerely learn the Principles, the degree to which you expend your efforts, the depth to which you understand these Principles, and the regularity with which you practice and apply them in your everyday life.

The **E**: The two relaxation **E**xercises are designed to give you the ability to calm your mind and body regardless of how stressful your circumstances are. When practiced daily, these exercises will help your mind and body relax and de-stress. These relaxation exercises are especially useful when you feel extremely stressed and your mind just can't deal with it and you can't think clearly. Doing these exercises will slow down your thoughts, halt your restlessness, relax your body, calm your mind, and soothe your whole being. Once you regain control, you will be able to think clearly and make any further decisions necessary.

The **T**: The calming **T**echnique (that you will be given to practice every day for at least 20 minutes, preferably in the morning) will strengthen your willpower, improve your concentration, and halt the restless thoughts in your mind. The end result is a peaceful and joyful state of mind, when you practice this technique regularly.

Although each of the components of the P-E-T System act through a different mechanism, the final outcome you derive from practicing them is the same: peace of mind and happiness. As you practice the P-E-T System every day, you will reap the benefits, and they will be evident in your daily life.

In the following chapters, you will discover each element of *The P-E-T System of Stress-Free Living* and how to integrate them into your daily life.

DR. CALM'S PRESCRIPTION

1 The components of P-E-T are: three **Principles**, two **Exercises**, one **Technique**.

2 Mastering the P-E-T System maximizes your ability to access and maintain a calm, peaceful mind.

3 With a calm mind, you can discover solutions to problems and enjoy success in life.

CHAPTER 15

The Three Principles: The Golden Key to Stress Freedom

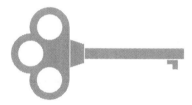

Mind, Thought, and Consciousness are the three principles that enable us to acknowledge and respond to existence. It is through these three components that all psychological mysteries are unfolded. All three are universal constants that can never change and never be separated. All three elements are the lifeline to our very existence.

They are what I call the psychological trinity.

~ **SYDNEY BANKS,** *The Missing Link*

Sydney Banks and the Three Principles

In 1973, Sydney Banks, an ordinary working man, had a profound insight into the Principles that underlie the foundation for human experience. With that new understanding, he noticed that life started becoming simpler. A natural joy started emanating from within, and peace of mind became a norm rather than a sporadic experience. Over time, his neighbors, strangers, and people from all over the world started seeking his help to solve the problems of their lives. They often found his simple wisdom to be practical and life changing. Even psychiatrists, psychotherapists, doctors, and other health professionals started learning from this humble man who had little formal education.

> The Principles are part and parcel of you already. You just have to realize them.

This tells us something—to achieve peace of mind and happiness, you don't have to learn rocket science. Whether you are a plumber, janitor, doctor, engineer, actor, celebrity, teacher, or a person with no formal education at all, these Principles are so simple that anyone can learn and understand them if you are sincere in your efforts. In fact, the Principles are part and parcel of you already. You just have to realize them. It does not matter where you are in your life's journey, these Principles will help you. These Principles are universal; thus, they are applicable under all circumstances.

When you listen with your heart and not your intellect, you will truly understand the Principles.

Don't memorize these Principles. Instead, understanding them deeply with your heart and mind—for what they are and how they underlie our human experience—will positively transform your life. When the understanding of these Principles dawns on you, stress escapes from the backdoors of your mind. Peace, joy, and contentment find their way back to your heart. This seemingly complex life becomes simple. You will start appreciating the profound nature of this creation. You will become an epicenter of joy and, slowly, people notice—you become a positive influence. Your life moves forward effortlessly in a miraculous way. All these positive experiences in life will help you develop faith in yourself and the natural balance and justice of this creation. Hope becomes not a momentary spark but a sustained light that shows the way out of even the deepest and darkest of troubles. Allow my and other people's positive life experiences using these Principles stand as a bridge of trust until you develop your own positive experiences using them. So, are you ready to enter a stress-free world?

The Difference between Universal Principles and Human-made Rules

Three Principles are universally applicable, regardless of circumstances, country, creed, gender, age, and all other variables. Human-made laws and rules are conditional and have limited applicability. Let's take the speed limit as an example. Currently, the maximum speed in the state of New York is 65 mph. But in Texas, it goes up to 85 mph. At one time, the New York State speed limit was only 55 mph, during the energy crisis of the 1970s. Do you see how the applicability of human-made laws changes with time, space, and circumstances? Although some of these laws are practical and are applicable under specific conditions, they are not universally applicable. However, universal principles like gravity are timeless and changeless. They are like the true north in a compass. We can use them as guideposts that lead us to the right destination.

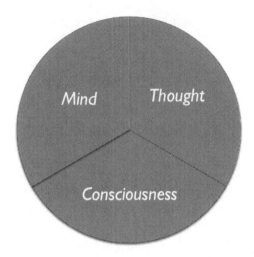

Figure 15.1. The Three Principles

The Three Principles are Universal

The Three Principles are such universal principles. They are not confined to one country, religion, sect, or community. They are applicable to all people in this world. They are self-evident and a part of our human nature. (In this book, whenever I use the term *Principle* with a capital *P*, it means it is universally applicable to all people in all situations.) Like the principle of gravity existed before and after Newton discovered it, these Three Principles have been there before and after Sydney Banks discovered them. Although different people during different periods of time on this earth have expressed them in different ways, the core Principles remain the same. These universal principles of mental well-being were organized under the name "Three Principles" by Sydney Banks.

Mind, Thought, and Consciousness (see Figure 15.1)

The Three Principles are *Mind, Thought,* and *Consciousness.*
The *Mind* is the intelligent energy behind all life. *Mind* is the

power that makes *life* possible. It is the power of *Mind* that creates, and sustains, everything in the universe.

Thought is the intelligent force that directs you through life and helps navigate it. It is rudder of life. It takes you where you want to go.

Consciousness is the intelligent power that gives us the ability to be aware of our experiences in life.

We are all born with these three divine gifts. Your destiny depends on how you use these gifts.

The Mind

Your mind can be compared to the engine of a car. A car does not move forward if the engine malfunctions; likewise, your life will not move forward if your mind is dysfunctional. For the car, the engine is the source of all energy and power. For your life, your mind is the source of all energy and power. You rely on the power of your mind to do well in life.

Let's say you've just purchased that dream car you always wanted. Excited, you get into the driver's seat, turn on the ignition, and press down on the gas pedal, expecting it to jump forward and ride smoothly. But the car does not move. What the heck? You press down harder on the gas pedal. But the car still doesn't start. Instead, a warning sign flashes on your dashboard: engine malfunction. Frustrated, you get out of the car, kick it hard, and then cry out loud with pain. Kicking the car won't fix your problem but fixing the engine would. Much like the dysfunctional car, you won't have a smooth ride in life if your mind isn't working properly. Just as you have to maintain your car's engine, you have to keep yourself in a good state of mind.

Thought

> Now, let us say the engine is in perfect condition. You decide to go for a drive. You sit in the car, grab hold of the steering wheel, and are ready to go. You push down on the gas pedal and try to steer the car out of your driveway—to no avail. The steering wheel is rigid as a rock; it won't move. You can't even steer your way out of the driveway. For you to drive the car to your desired destination, you need a functional steering wheel. In the same way, wherever you want to go in your life, your thoughts steer you there.

Your thoughts act like a steering wheel, taking you wherever you want to go in life. You can steer yourself either to a state of positive feelings (i.e., a peaceful and joyful state of mind) or a state of negative feelings (i.e., an unhappy and distressed mind), depending on where you focus your thoughts. Changing your state of mind is as simple as turning the steering wheel. You have a choice: you can turn your focus to good thoughts that lead to good feelings, or you can dwell on bad thoughts that lead to bad feelings.

You can drive your car either to a good neighborhood or a bad neighborhood; likewise, you can direct your life to either good destinations or bad destinations. It all depends on deciding where you want to go. Sometimes, you may accidentally end up in a bad neighborhood, but that doesn't mean that you have to stay there forever. In the same way, every now and then you may find yourself in a negative state. That does not mean you have to stay there. Simply turn back to a positive state in the same way you turn your car away from a bad neighborhood. It is really that simple.

Remember: You are the power behind the steering wheel of your thoughts. The choice is yours. At every turn of life, you have a choice: to turn toward good or to turn toward bad. The more you practice making this choice, the easier it will become to navigate yourself to positive states. It is by using the power of thought that we *create* good or bad in our lives, that we *feel* happy or sad, and that we *live* peacefully or miserably. So, take control of your life *now* by taking control of your thought power! Realize that you are the creator of your thoughts and thus your destiny!

Consciousness

Now your engine is in perfect working condition and so the steering wheel. You finally drive your car out of the driveway onto the street. But because of a snowstorm last night, the windshield and windows of the car are frosty, and you can't see clearly. Your car has a powerful engine, a power steering wheel that is responsive, and the best GPS in the world, but you are still stuck in your driveway because you can't see a single thing through your windshield and windows. You need to clear the frost so that you can see the world around, know where you are going, and enjoy the journey. If you cannot see through that windshield, you cannot have a safe journey.

In the same way, while you navigate life, you should be able to see where you are going. It is your consciousness that acts as a window through which you see your life experiences. It informs you where you are, what is happening within and around you, and whether you are at a desirable place in your life. *Consciousness* is the awareness of your life and its experiences. It gives you the ability to enjoy life's experiences.

Clouded consciousness is dangerous. If your awareness levels are low, you carry a high risk of making mistakes and getting into the accidents of life called *problems*. As your consciousness or awareness levels (of self and others) increase, you gain a better understanding of life. Life becomes more enjoyable. Grace flows into your life miraculously. The difficulties of life become easier or disappear altogether. Positive attitude and pleasant demeanor become your new way of living.

Yet, you may ask, what clears the fogginess of your consciousness? Calmness is the cleanser of your consciousness. As you become calmer and calmer, your consciousness becomes clearer and clearer. In that clarity, you see things as they are and understand them as they are meant to be.

Your Peace of Mind Is Just One Step Away

Regardless of how difficult your circumstances are, understand that your peace of mind is just one step away. All it takes is that one A-ha! moment, that one realization, for your mind to be set back to its default state—that is, peace of mind. If you are open to that possibility, seek the right knowledge, and sincerely make an effort toward that goal, you will succeed. I can vouch for this because I, myself, experienced such an awakening when my understanding of the Principles was rudimentary. See the following real-life example.

Many years ago, when I was in deep distress, I went to see my professor who was teaching resiliency and stress prevention at the university. She listened to me carefully and handed me some reading material and a CD. I walked back home, hoping to find solutions for the deep crisis I was in. At that time, I did not know how to solve my problem. So I couldn't help but sit and worry about it. Initially, I was skeptical whether the learning material would help me. However, I did not have any other solution. So I decided I'd give it a try. As I started listening to the CD, halfway through, something suddenly shifted in me. It seemed as if all my restless and worried thoughts were sucked out and a vacuum was created inside. I didn't understand what it was at that time, but a sense of peace started pouring from within. A few minutes later, I started feeling joyful.

I thought, "How is it possible to feel at peace all of a sudden when only minutes ago I was in deep distress and my thoughts were racing at a million miles per second? How can I feel joyful when I am in the middle of a deep crisis? No way. Something is wrong with me."

I picked up the phone and called my professor. Luckily, she answered. I quickly explained this strange experience to her.

She listened carefully and clarified what had happened to me in a matter-of-fact voice, "That's what happens when you understand these Principles. Your mind goes back to its default setting—peace and joy. There is nothing to be surprised about. It's quite natural."

I thought, "Wow! I have to study more about this," and I did.

An important point to notice here is that when I had that profound experience, I barely scratched the surface of these Principles. So, it does not take years, months, weeks, or even days to create that powerful shift within. It can happen today. It can happen this moment! Over the years, I have had many such profound experiences and insights. Now, whenever I feel stressed, I simply go back to my understanding of the Principles and peace follows.

The Transition from Stress to Peace Can be Effortless

Your ultimate goal is to strongly anchor yourself in a peaceful and joyful state of mind. A calm mind is the source of endless wisdom that harbors the solutions to all your problems. Once you learn to keep yourself calm and composed and make it a strong habit, nothing can shake you up. Of course, life will throw challenges at you every now and then, but if you know how to handle them gracefully, you don't have to be afraid of those challenges. You will remain unruffled no matter what!

The more you understand the Three Principles, the more you will be able to experience peace and joy; the transition from stress to peace happens effortlessly. The beauty of these Principles is that they are universal and thus are applicable in all kinds of situations at all times in our lives. The following example demonstrates that.

> Many years ago, when I was not at all aware of the Three Principles, I used to live in a stressful state of mind most of the time. When bad things happened to me, I always found a reason to blame the circumstances or the people around me. I lived like that for many years. For me, life at that time was a pendulum of emotions, moving from one extreme to another. I was completely ignorant of the fact that it was I who was swinging that pendulum of emotions from one extreme to another. I was the perpetuator of my emotions. How strange!
>
> When I was upset or angry about something, I used to shut the door of my room and find my favorite self-help book to read. After a while, I would emerge with a solution, all excited and relieved. Over the years, this happened again and again so many times, and I could not

understand how it was possible that every time I read a book I got answers to the dilemmas of my life. I did not know the answer to that question at that time.

Later, after many years, in retrospect, I understood that the answers were coming from my inner wisdom, and the book acted like a conduit to calm down my restless thoughts. As soon as I withdrew myself from the problem to relax and enjoy reading the book, my mind had a chance to calm down. In that calmness, I found clarity and focus to solve the problem at hand. Not to say that the knowledge gained from good books is not helpful, but it was my inner wisdom that automatically kicked in and showed me what path to follow. If it were just the books that were the source of the solutions, all people who read books would become free of problems. I gave as gifts many of the books I read to my friends and family members, but to my dismay, very few of them found them as helpful and fascinating as I did. I used to get upset with them, "What's wrong with you? Can't you see how wonderful this book is? It has all the solutions to your problems!" I didn't realize that the real source of the solution to my problems was my calm mind.

Finally, I got it. I said to myself, "It is me and my own innate wisdom that channeled the knowledge in the book to find a solution for my problems." This reasoning also explained why I used to feel calm after reading suspenseful and thrilling fiction novels. This is another example proving that it is not the content of the book but the art of taking your mind away from worrisome thinking and giving it a chance to relax that is the real reason for accessing your inner peace and wisdom.

The Real Reason Behind Your Peace of Mind

You might find it helpful to go for a walk, sit quietly in a park, dance, hike, listen to music, or listen to the calming roar of the ocean. I used to find them helpful, too. But the truth is it is not the beach or park that is giving you peace of mind, it is the quieting of the restless thoughts in your mind that gives you that peace.

> It is not the beach or park that is giving you peace of mind, it is the quieting of the restless thoughts in your mind that gives you that peace.

After all these years, when I remember how I recovered from so many stressful situations, I marvel at how powerfully resilient the human spirit is, even in those days when I was not aware of these Principles. But when I learned these Principles, peace and joy became more of a norm than an exception.

Unwrap Your Divine Gifts

To reap the benefits of life, we need to unwrap the three divine gifts of Mind, Thought, and Consciousness. The power of these Three Principles will propel you toward a happy, peaceful, and productive life. You will see a profound, positive transformation.

DR. CALM'S PRESCRIPTION

1. ✓ You don't have to be a scholar to understand the Three Principles. They are simple, straightforward, and easy to understand. All you have to do is be sincere and listen with your heart. When you understand them for what they are, your life will be transformed.

2. ✓ The Three Principles are universal. Thus, they are applicable in all situations of life, regardless of time and circumstance. They are secretly operating throughout the universe whether you know about them or not. The deeper your understanding of the Three Principles and your alignment with them, the simpler and more enjoyable your life becomes.

3. ✓ The *Mind* is the intelligent energy that creates and sustains all life. The *Mind* is like the engine of a car; it's the source of all power. Without the engine of the mind, the car of life does not move forward. So, keep your mind healthy.

4. ✓ *Consciousness* is the intelligent, all-knowing power that helps you experience and be aware of your life. Our *Consciousness* is like the windshield of a car. As you drive, you see where you are going through the windshield.

5. ✓ *Thought* is an intelligent force that directs you through life and helps navigate it. *Thought* is like the steering wheel of the car. The steering wheel of *Thought* helps you to steer your way to beautiful—or the most horrible—feelings in life.

6. ✓ You are the power behind your thoughts, and you have the power to steer your life to either a happy destination or a miserable one.

7. ✓ Your ultimate goal is to strongly anchor yourself in a peaceful and joyful state of mind. The Three Principles help you do that effortlessly.

CHAPTER 16

The Two Exercises: The Golden Art of Letting Go

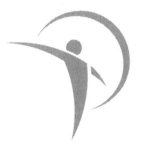

*Letting go of your attachment to thoughts
is the only true way out of stress.*

Letting Go—The Only Way Out of Stress

A major problem we all face is the difficulty of letting go of negative thoughts. It feels like your mind has a propensity to cling to negative thoughts. Most of your stress would be gone if you could allow those thoughts to pass.

Imagine that you are driving to work, and on the way, you see

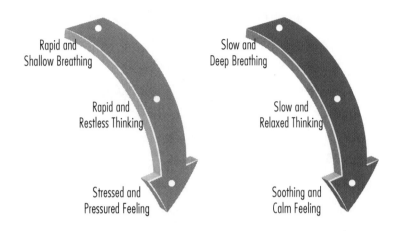

Figure 16.1. The Relationship between Breathing, Thinking, and Feeling

an accident. You don't stop. You see that the police and the EMTs are taking care of it. What happens if all the drivers passing by notice the accident and pull over? There would then be severe congestion on the highway. The accident victims might be more difficult to reach. Likewise, if you obstruct the flow of thoughts on the highway of your mind, it causes thought congestion and leads to stress. To clear that stress, all you have to do is to ignore negative thoughts and move on. Negative thoughts are accidents in your mind. Leave them alone and they will disappear. By doing so, the traffic of thoughts in your mind will automatically return to normal flow, and everything will fall into place.

As Breathing Is for the Body, Thinking Is for the Mind

Negative thoughts are tenacious. Sometimes, however hard you try, you find them stuck to you. During those times, it helps to practice thought detachment, using relaxation exercises that slow down your breathing. Breathing exercises are easy to practice and have a powerful, calming effect on your mind by slowing down your thoughts.

The Ancient Connection between Your Breathing and Your Thoughts (see Figure 16.1)

Your breathing and thinking are closely related to each other. Rapid and shallow breathing often leads to rapid and shallow thinking, too. When you breathe rapidly, your body feels stressed. There is increased demand on your bodily organs. Lactic acid and other toxins accumulate and cause fatigue. In the same way, when your mind is racing fast with restless thoughts, you will feel mentally stressed, tired, and irritated. This leads to mental fatigue. As you rest your body when fatigued, so you also need to regularly rest your mind to avoid overuse and fatigue.

Knowing this connection between breathing and thinking, ancient saints of India discovered breathing exercises that calm the body and mind. *Because thoughts are subtle and hard to control, an indirect way of controlling thoughts is to regulate breathing.* When you breathe slowly and deeply, your thinking automatically slows down, too. It rests your body; your mind feels relaxed and calm.

The following are the two foundational relaxation exercises of the P-E-T System. You can build upon them and vary them according to circumstances and need. When you feel you are stressed, practice either one or both of them for a strong, calming effect. I recommend devoting 5 to 10 minutes to each exercise. However, in certain circumstances, when a longer length is not possible, even 1 or 2 minutes will produce a marked result if done with complete focus. Many times during my life, I have used these relaxation exercises to great benefit.

Exercise 1: Complete Mind-Body-Breath Relaxation

1. Lie down or sit back in an easy chair; completely relax both your mind and body. Just let go of everything—every thought, idea, limitation, pain, every past event or future worry, every feeling,

just about everything that could possibly arise in your mind—
and just relax completely and ease into your body and mind.

2. Breathe deeply and release your breath slowly. Again, breathe
deeply and release slowly. Do it a few times—possibly for the
next few minutes. You feel your body and mind relaxing. Just
ease into your breathing.

3. Let your breathing take a natural rhythm and follow it. Your
breathing will slow down and will become very enjoyable and
relaxing. Ease into it. Let it be. Let nothing bother you at this
time. You are alone. You are free. You are enjoying yourself.

- Remind yourself that you have no limitations other than
those you impose on yourself. As you breathe, notice that
you can take only one breath at a time. Observe that one
breath. Be in that moment, be in that breath completely.

- Then release the breath slowly, naturally. Be completely with
it from the beginning to the end of the exhale. Observe it.
Then let the next breath in. And continue the cycle. As you
continue to do this, your breathing will slow down, your
thoughts will slow down, and your awareness levels will rise.

- Whenever you lose the flow of observing your breathing,
remind yourself that you can only take one breath at a time,
that you can only either breathe in or breathe out; you can't
do both at once. Then why jump forward and think about
the next breath and the next moment? Stay with the breath
and stay in the moment.

4. As you relax and ease into this state, you will feel all the restlessness in your body and mind completely dissolve. If you
still feel a bit of restlessness, continue to ease into your breathing. Just let it be. If you want to, observe your breathing as it
naturally happens.

5. Doing this exercise for 5 to 10 minutes is usually sufficient to completely relax you, but if you feel like you need to do it longer, that's

fine, too. But within the first 5 minutes, you may notice yourself falling into a sleeplike state in which you are deeply relaxed.

6. Rest there as long as you feel like before you return to your normal self. You will wake up feeling refreshed and rejuvenated. Now your mind is clear, and you can carry on with your life and your daily activities.

Exercise 2: Relaxation on the Go—A Flowing Meditation on Your Thoughts

1. Every day as you walk, sit, or engage in any other activity, take time to notice your breathing and your thoughts. You can do this any number of times during the day.

2. Remind yourself that your true nature is peace of mind. Remind yourself that your joy is within and is independent of all external conditions.

3. Remember, it is your thoughts that create your reality. Whatever situation that you are seeing now is just a momentary reality. That momentary reality will have to pass and, in the next moment, a new momentary reality will emerge. And so on it goes.

4. Any reality is real to you only as long as you focus on it. The moment you let go of the previous thought, the next thought will come forward, creating a new momentary reality.

5. So, your reality essentially changes from moment to moment as you move along your thought train, choosing the thoughts you want to entertain.

6. As you choose positive and constructive thoughts, your reality will mold itself in that same way. If you choose to focus on negative and destructive thoughts, your reality will change to be the same. It is entirely up to you what thoughts you want to entertain.

7. To be able to choose your thoughts—and, thus, your reality— it is important to be as self-aware as you can to be able to consciously choose the direction you want to take in life. This exercise develops that self-awareness.

DR. CALM'S PRESCRIPTION

1 ✓ Negative thoughts can be tenacious. There are times you will try with all of your might but find it very difficult to let go of negative thoughts. In these situations, breathing exercises can come to your rescue.

2 ✓ Breathing exercises are easy to use and have a powerful, calming effect on your mind. As your breathing slows down, your thinking automatically slows down, too.

3 ✓ The mind is subtle and difficult to control. But your breathing is more easily observable, thus making it an indirect tool to controlling your mind.

4 ✓ Do not force your breathing to slow down. Just observe the natural flow of your breath going in and out. Automatically, it will slow down. If your mind wanders to something else besides your breathing, bring it gently back. With practice, you will get better at this.

5 ✓ When you are totally relaxed, your breathing and your thoughts almost become unnoticeable, creating a calming effect on your body and mind. Remain in this state as long as you can. If your mind wanders, resume the breathing exercise again. Remember: The goal is not the exercise itself but reaching a state of total relaxation and remaining there.

6 ✓ Another way to let go of negative thoughts is to remind yourself of your true nature. Remind yourself that you are more than your circumstances. You are not your thoughts either. You are the creator of your thoughts.

7 ✓ Know that thoughts are transient and only create transient realities. Beneath the superficial tumultuous waves of thoughts, your *Real Self* remains unperturbed.

CHAPTER 17

The One Technique: The Golden Gateway to Deep Calmness

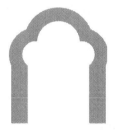

If there is only one habit that you have to develop for achieving great success and happiness in life, it is the habit of attaining deep calmness.

The Power of Habit

In the garden of life, the seeds of thoughts sown into the soil of your mind innocently grow into the powerful trees of habits. You have a choice whether to sow the seeds of good thoughts or the

173

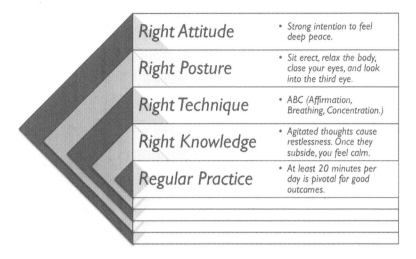

Right Attitude	• Strong intention to feel deep peace.
Right Posture	• Sit erect, relax the body, close your eyes, and look into the third eye.
Right Technique	• ABC (Affirmation, Breathing, Concentration.)
Right Knowledge	• Agitated thoughts cause restlessness. Once they subside, you feel calm.
Regular Practice	• At least 20 minutes per day is pivotal for good outcomes.

Figure 17.1. The Key Determinants of Successful Meditation

weeds of bad thoughts in your mind. Thoughts when persistently repeated, get solidified into strong habits. These habits guide your life to your destiny. *Habits have the power to either propel you to the sky of success or drag you to the abyss of failure.*

If you have built good habits, your life will be on a roll. With the power of strong habits, even difficult tasks become easy. If you build bad habits, even easy goals become difficult. Bad habits obstruct you from achieving your goals and thus become obstacles to your success.

Calmness Is a Habit

Calmness is a habit and so is stress. You may say that it is difficult to remain calm and there is always something to disturb your peace of mind. Being calm is difficult because your habit of being restless is stronger than the habit of being calm. Since childhood, your environment has conditioned you to be restless. In this society, few people talk about the importance of calmness. Rarely, we are taught how to be calm. *Without proper guidance, the human mind follows the path of least resistance and sulks*

in restlessness rather than building the beneficial habit of calmness.
Most people are not even aware that they are restless, and they live
in that restless state of mind all their life thinking that it is normal.
I did, too, until I discovered the power of calmness!

You may be thinking, "How am I going to arrest the restless
monkey mind? Isn't it too hard to do that? Is it even possible?"
Yes! It is possible. The good news is the more you practice being
calm, the easier it gets to arrest restlessness. With the right attitude,
knowledge, and technique, it doesn't take much time to attain a
state of deep calmness. Daily practice of the technique described
below will help you anchor yourself in the habit of calmness. And,
one day, your habit of calmness will become so strong, even the
pandemonium of crashing worlds will not unsettle you!

The Right Technique at the Right Time

More than ten years ago, when I was experiencing extreme restlessness, one of my friends introduced me to a meditation technique. I
had tried meditation before but it did not work.
So, I was initially skeptical. However, my need
to calm down was so great that I was ready to
try anything that could help me. *Necessity is the
mother of motivation!* I quickly read the step-
by-step instructions on how to practice meditation. I sat down in a quiet room and practiced
the technique. I did not know what to expect but I nevertheless sat
there for the next 10–15 minutes. Although my mind was restless,
my effort was sincere. When I opened my eyes, I felt different. I
knew something had changed in me. I felt calm. The thoughts that
were bothering me for many days disappeared and were replaced by
a subtle but clearly noticeable stream of positive feelings. My mind
became impervious to the difficulties and the negativity that enveloped me. All in all, I felt hopeful and elated.

Necessity is
the mother
of motivation!

As I went on to carry out my daily activities, things started happening effortlessly in my life. People around me were nicer to me and more helpful than usual. I came back home and started reflecting on my day, I realized I had an excellent day, considering the grave situation I was in. As I continued to practice meditation more and more, I noticed that my life was on a roll. Along with feeling a deep sense of security from within, an intuitive inner voice guided me to the right opportunities at the right time, again and again. The end result was that in the three months following my first meditation, I was completely out of trouble and was carried to the perfect place that would unfold some of the most beautiful moments in my life.

> Hard work and perseverance — when compounded by the power of calmness — catapult you effortlessly to the shores of success and happiness.

In my mind, I developed a strong conviction that, *in the sea of life, hard work and perseverance—when compounded by the power of calmness—catapult you effortlessly to the shores of success and happiness.* Time and again, this truth was proved right in my life. Thereafter, I never looked back and never stopped meditating. I kept exploring more deeply the ocean of meditation. After much research, practice, and experience, I designed the unique technique that can be practiced by anyone regardless of their creed, race, religion, gender, nation, or any other identification.

The ABC Calming Technique

Use the ABC (affirmation, breathing, concentration) technique below for your benefit. You will reap the greatest benefit when you practice it regularly every day for at least 20 minutes, giving it your complete and undivided attention.

Some important points to remind yourself before attempting the technique:

1. The good news is all problems have a solution.
2. The key to finding solutions to problems in life is calmness.
3. When you become deeply calm, automatically your inner wisdom comes forth and shows you the solution to your problems.
4. When you need to find a solution to a problem, deepen your state of calmness to the point where all restless thoughts subside. Then you will be left with deep peace and joy emanating from within.
5. In that state, you will find guidance and very clearly see what needs to be done. The Universe or God or greater power—whatever you want to call it—that force will come to your aid and rearrange your life situations to facilitate natural harmony in your life.
6. If you learn to access that calm state of mind all the time, you not only solve problems easily, you will also prevent them.
7. Practice this technique every day for the next 20 days, and great benefits will follow.

General Rules

1. Get up early in the morning, preferably before 6 a.m. (as early as you can, depending on your schedule).
2. Take a bath or shower.
3. Find a quiet place where you won't be disturbed.
4. Practice the calming technique for at least 20 minutes.
5. The peak point of your practice is when you feel all the thoughts in your mind just disappear and you feel deep sense of peace (when you are there, you will know it—you will feel it).
6. Stay in that feeling of deep peace for as long as possible.
7. Conclude your practice and carry on with your daily

activities. Try to hold on to that peace within and carry it everywhere you go.

The ABC Technique has the following three components:

1. **A**ffirmation: With deep attention, say to yourself, "I am calm" or "I am peace" or "I am joy."
2. **B**reathing: Take a few deep breaths (10–15 deep breaths), inhaling deeply and exhaling slowly. Be aware of the pause between inhalation and exhalation. If you can maintain the inhalation, the pause, and outgoing breath each to a count of 10 to 15, it will be most beneficial.
3. **C**oncentration: Close your eyes and concentrate. Focus attention on the point between your two eyebrows. (See below for complete instructions.)

Affirmations with deep attention work because:

- Your attention is directed away from restless thoughts and that energy is instead used to focus on something positive and calming. The momentum built up by your restless thoughts dies away and is replaced by a calm feeling.
- We become whatever we focus upon. If we focus on negative thoughts, we tend to become negative. If we focus on positive thoughts, we certainly see more positivity around us. If we intend to become calm, we will become calm.

> Please do not mistake intention plus deep attention with controlling thoughts.

Please do not mistake intention plus deep attention with *controlling* thoughts. Here, you are not controlling your thoughts. You are merely focusing on one thought (of becoming calm) and letting other thoughts subside. Sometimes, letting go of worrisome thoughts happens easily and naturally. When it does not happen easily, you need techniques to help you. Instead of fighting the thoughts, simply divert your awareness and energy to any other thought that is positive, *neutral,* and calming. That will bring peace.

However, do not focus on anything exciting. That will make you more restless. For example, if you imagine your ideal partner or a beautiful vacation destination, it initially might create a positive feeling, but if you continue to focus on it, it may lead to an obsession and a need to possess it; this, in turn, can lead to restlessness, as you keep thinking in your mind how to achieve what you want and whether you can achieve it, and so on. *The whole purpose of the calming exercise will then be in vain.*

The easiest and surest way to practice the technique is to choose a simple, neutral, and positive affirmation like calmness, peace, and joy. Love can also be used, although I prefer to avoid the word "love" because it means very different things to different people, which can lead to confusion.

With this effort, your mind immediately recognizes your intention to be calm and will stimulate the parts of your brain that assist you with this goal.

Specific Instructions

1. Sit straight either on a chair or on the floor. Make sure that your spine is erect, and your chin parallel to the ground. Keep your hands, legs, and body relaxed. Do not lean against the back of the chair or the wall. If you have to lean against something to support your back, that is okay in these preliminary stages. But, where possible, avoid it.

2. Close your eyes. Take your index finger and touch the point between your eyebrows. That's your "spiritual eye," or "third eye." That's the point of super consciousness. *Mentally* focus on that point. Don't try too hard to focus; stay relaxed. (After a while, you will learn how to locate your spiritual eye mentally and there will be no need to

use your index finger to touch and locate it physically. This comes with practice.)

3. Now, do the affirmation (the *A* component) as described above for 2 to 3 minutes. This will remind you of your true nature and the true purpose of doing this technique. Then do the breathing (the *B* component) as described above for 2 to 3 minutes. Doing the *A* and *B* components will prepare you to practice deep concentration and attain deep calmness. Then start concentrating deeply (the *C* component).

4. Initially, your eyes tend to drift away from the spiritual eye because they are habituated to restlessness, as your mind is habituated to restless thoughts. There is a direct connection between the restlessness of your thoughts and the restlessness of your eyes. Once your eyes calm down and stay focused on the spiritual eye, automatically your thoughts will slow down, too. Likewise, once you learn to calm your thoughts, your eyes will lose their restlessness and will be able to calmly focus on anywhere you want with deep concentration. It takes practice to achieve such one-pointed concentration. With time, you will achieve it. Sometimes, this may happen right away and sometimes it may take a little effort.

5. Every time your mental focus drifts away from the spiritual eye, gently bring it back. As you try to keep your focus on the spiritual eye, thoughts may restlessly dance in your mind and try to distract you. Don't let them. Regardless of what kind of thoughts they are, know that it does not matter; do not focus on them. Let them pass, as unattended thoughts will surely pass. Know that you are not your thoughts. Know that all thoughts are transient, and each thought creates only an illusory reality that is going to disappear when the thought passes. So, just let any thought that comes to your mind pass. Keep your focus on the spiritual eye.

6. To help keep your focus on the spiritual eye, I recommend

chanting a neutral word or mantra. When your mind focuses on the mantra, it will more easily let go of the restless thoughts that are trying to distract you. With strong resolve and persistent concentration, keep focusing on the spiritual eye, and at some point in time, suddenly all the thoughts in your mind disappear as if they have been sucked out by a vacuum; that is, you will be in a calm state of mind. When that happens, and before a restless thought tries to disturb your mind again, stay there as long as you can. If you notice an uninvited thought coming back, ignore it, gently bring your attention back to the spiritual eye, and the restless thought will disappear. As you sink deeper into this calm state of mind, you will find great peace emanating from within and enveloping you from without.

7. Remain in this state as long as you can. Before you conclude your meditation session, before opening your eyes, if you would like to, ask for any problem in your life to be solved. Sometimes, the answer comes to you immediately; at other times, the answer will come to you as a deep insight while you are carrying out your activities during the day. This may happen all of a sudden when you are not actually thinking about the problem. Often, you experience things suddenly falling into place, people becoming nicer to you, and obstacles in your path to success disappearing. You will have a much smoother journey in life than people who don't meditate regularly.

The key to successful meditation is regularity (see Figure 17.1). The more often and longer you meditate, the greater your happiness and success will be.

Meditation: Differentiating the Myths from the Truth

Myth #1: Meditation is a Religious Practice

Truth: Meditation Is a Practical Tool, Not a Religious Practice

Many people think meditation is a religious practice. That's not true. You don't have to be of specific religion to practice meditation. People also say that meditation is a spiritual practice. I say that it is a spiritual practice for those who think it is spiritual and it is a practical tool for those who simply want a better life. Though there are obvious spiritual benefits due to meditation, you don't have to be spiritually inclined at all to practice it. You could be a spiritual novice, or even have no intention to tread on a spiritual path but you could still immensely benefit from meditation as it instills calmness, an antidote to stress.

Myth # 2: Meditation Makes You More Restless

Truth: Meditation Alleviates Restlessness and Improves Your Focus

Novice meditators may notice restlessness in their thoughts at first, giving them a false impression that they are becoming more restless. But, the truth is that meditation helps them calm down enough to notice how restless they are for the first time. But, as you continue your meditation, the restless thoughts slowly subside and eventually disappear totally. Meditation aids in developing deep concentration, great focus, and finally helps you achieve an absolutely still state of mind where there is not even a flicker of restless thought to disturb your tranquility. The deep peace and joy that abounds in that state is indescribable, but it can be felt by the meditator. It is often perceptible.

> Meditation aids in developing deep concentration, great focus, and an absolutely still state of mind.

People around you may notice you to be more cheerful and optimistic. You may find yourself being able to carry out multiple tasks at once, with less effort. You will be more energetic and less distracted. The end result is less stress, more joy, and better performance, both at work and home.

Myth #3: Sitting Long in a Meditative Posture Means You Have Meditated Well

Truth: It is not Meditative Posture Itself but Attaining a Calm State of Mind that Signifies Whether You Have Meditated Truly or Not

The act of sitting in a meditative posture itself doesn't mean you are meditating. There are people who sit in a meditative posture for hours and yet they never truly experience meditation. You may sit in a meditative posture for hours but if your mind remains restless, you will not experience the deeply peaceful meditative state of mind. Often, it is incorrect technique that prevents many from finding a true meditative experience. It's like playing tennis using the wrong technique. You could practice tennis for years by yourself but you may not progress well because you lack the right technique. With the right coach teaching you the right technique, you quickly improve your game. The same is also true for meditation. Learn the right technique and you will see the results immediately.

Myth #4 Meditation is Something You Do

Truth: Meditation is Not Just an Act; It is the Experience

Meditation is both a noun and verb. When you say, "I do meditation," meditation is a verb—the act of sitting in a meditative posture and practicing a meditative technique. When you say, "I am in meditation," it is a noun which means you are in a state of meditation—an absolutely still and calm state of mind. Often, people confuse the noun meditation with the verb meditation. It's important to differentiate. Just because you have spent 30 minutes practicing a meditative technique doesn't necessarily mean that you have attained a meditative state of mind. All that you do prior to attaining a meditative state of mind is called pre-meditation. Often that pre-meditative effort is needed to attain a meditative state of mind. However, some people may be able to put themselves in a meditative state of mind in no time and without using any technique. Often, that happens when you have been a longtime practitioner. Sometimes, that may happen to you even without any effort, which is called *spontaneous meditation*. But in general, the more you practice the greater your chances to have a successful meditation.

Myth #5: It Takes Years to Benefit from Meditation

Truth: Even a Little Practice Can Bring a Big Change

The motivating truth for beginning meditators is that even a little bit of effort to meditate is beneficial and with regular practice soon you will see perceptible positive changes in life. Once you experience deep calmness and the good feelings that come along with it, your mind will seek more of it. That automatically makes practicing meditation easier and more enjoyable.

Every day I see many hardworking people struggling to succeed. They feel that their hard work has fallen short of bringing them the success and happiness they deserve. I can't help but notice that their restlessness is what is preventing them from having real success in life. If you start practicing the technique described, it will dissolve restlessness and bring you success in life.

DR. CALM'S PRESCRIPTION

1   No matter how stressed you are and how difficult your situation is your peace of mind is just a moment away. You might experience that deeply peaceful state at any moment.

2   Anyone can find peace of mind instantly. But to remain in that state takes practice. Calmness is a habit, and the more you practice it, the better you get at it. One day, you will be so calm that even the most chaotic circumstances cannot distract you. Nothing can derail you in this state.

3   Your success with the ABC Calming Technique lies in regularity. Do it every day. Allot at least 20 minutes to practicing the technique, no matter what. In the same way that you eat, drink, and sleep every day, so should you practice the technique every day, and your life will become more wonderful than ever.

4   Sit erect, keep your spine straight, relax your body, and mentally concentrate on the spiritual eye. These are the four most important rules that you must strictly follow for the best results.

5   Practicing the technique in the early morning immediately after you wake up. That is the most beneficial time to practice meditation, as your mind is fresh and relaxed. Later during the day, your mind becomes preoccupied with your daily activities, making it more difficult to attain one pointed focus.

6   If you miss your morning practice, do it in the evening. If you completely miss it for a day, add 20 extra minutes to your practice the next day. But don't keep postponing.

7   The goal of the technique is to attain deep calmness. Once you attain that state, you can stop practicing the technique and stay in that calm state as long as possible. Enjoy it.

Moving Beyond Your Limitations

Part VI Objectives:

- Understand the nature of thought.
- Discover the Laws of Thought Mechanics.
- Realize the inside-out nature of this world.
- Redefine your perspective, resolve conflicts, and establish harmony.
- Deepen your presence and increase your awareness.
- Defy the past and build a brighter future.
- Improve your sleep.

CHAPTER 18

The Laws of Thought Mechanics

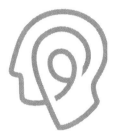

You are not your thoughts. You are that which is behind your thoughts. So, the negative thoughts you have about yourself are not the real you.

Knowing and Following the Right Laws of Life is the Difference Between Success and Failure

Your car is broken, and you take it to the mechanic. Because he knows how cars work, he fixes your car in minutes. It would have taken forever to fix it by yourself, if at all you were able to identify the problem in the first place. Likewise, if you understand thought mechanics, you can fix your mental world and run your life smoothly.*

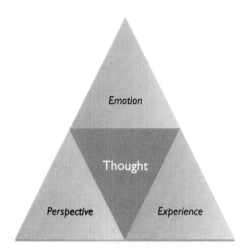

Figure 18.1. Perspective, Emotion, and Experience —
All Three Arise from Thought and Are Inseparable

Understanding how thoughts work will help access your mental well-being and live a stress-free life.

Newton's *laws of motion* are the three physical laws that laid the foundation for classical mechanics. Just as the laws of physical mechanics govern the physical world, the laws of thought mechanics govern our mental world. There are three laws of thought mechanics:

- **The First Law of Thought Mechanics:** Thoughts flow continuously in your mind. When you let them flow freely, you remain in a happy and relaxed state of mind.
- **The Second Law of Thought Mechanics:** Stagnated thoughts lead to a stressed state of mind. Attachment to thoughts leads to stagnation of thoughts.
- **The Third Law of Thought Mechanics:** The thoughts you focus on become your reality, and you perceive the reality you create.

The discussion below demonstrates these laws and makes it obvious that they are not a separate entity but an integral part of the Principle of Thought. These three laws are practically applicable for living a stress-free life. Before we start exploring these laws, let us understand first the nature of our thoughts and their relation to human experience.

Thought is a Universal Phenomenon and the Foundation of Human Experience

Thought is a divine gift; we all are born with the ability to think. *Thought is the link between the unmanifested and manifested aspects of life.* Without thought, no creation is possible, big or small. Without thought, this creation cannot be sustained. Without thought, nothing happens in this universe. Thought is a universal phenomenon. It is the missing link that determines your destiny.

Thoughts give you the ability to perceive. Out of that perception, your experience is born (see Figure 18.1). Without thoughts, there is no human experience. Without thoughts, you can't experience the senses of sight, smell, sound, touch, taste. You can't experience pain and pleasure. When you are deeply asleep, you are not aware of thoughts, and so you are not aware of the senses and experiences (unless you are dreaming). But you need thoughts even to dream. So, thought is the foundation of human experience.

Thought is the Fundamental Unit of the Creation

What an atom is for the physical world, thought is for the mental world. Thought is the quintessential and fundamental unit of our existence and our mental creation. As molecules, metals, nonmetals, cells, tissues, organs, and organisms can't exist without the fundamental unit called the atom, in the same way, without thoughts, our mental world cannot exist. *Without thought, there is no emotion, there are no ideas, there is no perception, and there is no mental world at all.* It is through thoughts that we perceive what we see, that we see what we perceive, and experience everything in this world. Without thought, there is neither pain nor pleasure. Without thought, there is neither love nor hatred. Thought is the link that connects the physical world to your mental world.

Your Physical World is a Direct Extension of Your Mental World

Every object that is created by humans, every invention, every discovery was possible only because of the human ability to think. Steve Jobs created the iPhone first in his mental world through thoughts, and then he created its physical counterpart. A house is built on the mental pillars of thoughts first before you get the blueprints. If the mental blueprint of the house is defective, then the house you build is also going to be faulty.

In the same way, *if your thoughts and thus your mental world are unpleasant, your physical world will also be unpleasant.* If you think bad thoughts, you will create a bad mental world, and that will manifest as bad outcomes in your physical world.

It is essential to recognize that *thought* is the fundamental unit of our lives, and without thought, our existence has no meaning. It is by using this power of thought that we create good or bad in our lives and as a result, live happily or miserably. So, take control of your life **now** by taking control of your thought power! Realize that you are the creator of your thoughts and thus your destiny!

The Origin of Your Thoughts

Did you ever wonder where your thoughts come from? How do they originate? How do they propagate? Who creates them? Do you think while you're sleeping?

Thoughts come from an Infinite Source, as thoughts themselves are infinite. Just for a moment, observe how thoughts come and go. Obviously, there are times when you actively create thoughts in your mind, but there are other times when thoughts appear in your mind out of nowhere. In one day, as many as fifty thousand thoughts pass through your mind. You are not actively thinking all of them; there are times when you are not even aware of your thoughts, and yet thoughts flow in the background of your mind. They flow continuously, all day and night, every day, every week, and every year—eternally.

The Universal Mind and the Personal Mind

Logically speaking, it makes sense that thoughts are being released continuously by an "Infinite Source." I call that Infinite Source, the Universal Mind—the source of all thoughts in the universe and so the thoughts in your mind. Our personal mind is a part of the Universal Mind. The following example demonstrates that.

Let us say you are a farmer in a small village that resides on the bank of a mighty river. You divert some of the water in the river into a small branch to irrigate your farm. That branch of the river can be compared to your personal mind. The mighty river can be compared to the Universal Mind. As the same water flows both in the river and its branches, the same thoughts flow in the Universal Mind and the personal mind. In a similar way that you have diverted the water from the river for your personal use, so do you personalize the thoughts flowing from the Universal Mind through your personal mind. This means that even your personal thoughts originate from the Universal Mind.

Ego Creates a Barrier between the Personal Mind and the Universal Mind

Ego separates your personal mind from the Universal Mind. When your ego prevails, your personal mind is operating. To the degree your ego prevails, your thoughts will be proportionately more selfish, isolated, and self-directed. It is the ignorance of your true nature that creates this artificial barrier called "ego" that gives you the illusion that your personal mind is separate from the Universal

Mind. To the degree you dissolve your ego, your thoughts become proportionately more selfless, liberating, and service oriented.

Dissolve the Ego and Harness the Power of the Infinite

Dissolving your ego is the way to attune yourself with the Universe. The thoughts that pass through your mind in that 'egoless state' are of a higher vibration, purity, positivity, and creativity. It's like running higher and higher up to the peak of the mountain where the stream of water originates. There, you get purer and clearer water in abundance than you would if you collected it farther downstream away from its original source. When that artificial barrier, your ego, dissolves completely, and when there is no more separation between the personal mind and the Universal Mind, then you will harness the power of the Universal Mind. You will be one with the power of the Infinite.

A Calm Mind Is the Doorway to Infinite Power

But what is the power that dissolves your ego and attunes your personal mind to the Universal Mind? The power of calmness puts you in touch with that universal source of power. When you are calm, the door of ego that separates your personal mind from the Universal Mind opens wide, allowing you to access that infinite power. To the degree that you are calm, it is to that degree the door opens. When your mind is absolutely still, without even a single flicker of a restless thought, the door dissolves completely, making your personal mind absolutely one with the Universal Mind.

A Free-Flowing State of Mind is Essential for Your Happiness

Thoughts flow in your mind continuously, as water flows in the river. Free-flowing water is naturally healthier and drinkable, unless you contaminate it; the same way, when thoughts flow freely in your mind, you will be in a naturally cheerful and peaceful state of mind. But when the flowing river is blocked, the water becomes stagnant, dirty, infested with bugs—unhealthy and undrinkable. Likewise, when you get attached to thoughts and block the free-flowing state of mind, it leads to stress. You regain your natural state of mind—becoming happy and peaceful—by letting your thoughts flow freely without getting attached to them.

Attachment to Thoughts Can Be Dangerous

Have you ever been bothered by a thought and couldn't shake it out of your mind? This has happened to me many times. What usually happens in these situations is that you keep thinking those worried thoughts, and they gather a momentum of their own, so much so that they intrude on everything you do despite your efforts to move on and focus on something else. Sometimes, this dysfunctional thinking affects you so much that you can't carry out your daily activities. I have seen such situations in my practice where people couldn't take their minds off specific thoughts and felt like they were acting on them against their will. In medical terminology, it's called *obsessive-compulsive disorder*. It ultimately affects all aspects of afflicted people's lives, including their relationships, job, finances, family life, and more.

Are You Obsessive-Compulsive?

Obsessive-compulsive disorder is an extreme form of thought attachment. Everyone experiences thought attachment to a certain degree, whether it is related to a person, object, deadline, goal, or something else. You are okay as long as you are able to withdraw your attention from them and move on to something else. The problem arises when those thoughts take over and you feel compulsive about them to the extent that you can't focus on anything else. The real problem comes when you think you must carry them out, otherwise you won't be happy—that's the birth of *conditional happiness*.

Thoughts Are Like Wild Horses—Don't Let Them Throw You Off and Drag You Around! (see Figure 18.2)

If you lose control of your thoughts, then thoughts take control of your life. It's like the rider who loses control of his horse. As long as you, the rider, controls the horse, you can ride wherever you want to. But the moment you lose control and the horse throws you off, you are in deep trouble. You may get injured. Sometimes, you may die if you are dragged down a cliff. The exact same thing happens when you are not in control of your thoughts and your thoughts gain momentum, take control over your life, and drag you down to bad feelings and bad actions. Eventually, you end up in a bad place in life, perhaps with an obsession for drugs, alcohol, smoking, sex, money, or some other dark desire.

Notice that all this happens because you have knowingly or unknowingly initiated some negative thoughts in your mind, got attached to them and then brooded over them, thus creating a momentum to the point where your thoughts gained a life of their own, dragging you down to bad places despite your own will. That is how all major problems in life start—through misuse of the power of thoughts—the dysfunctional, repetitive thinking program in your mind. So, do not initiate or encourage negative thinking!

Be the Master of Your Thoughts

So, what's the solution? The solution lies in realizing that you are the master of your thoughts. You have created them in the first place, and you have the ability to just stop thinking those undesirable thoughts. You can decide to let your thoughts flow by, simply realizing all thoughts are transient and they should flow naturally. Attachment to thoughts is what obstructs the flow. Whatever reality is being created by those thoughts is only real while those thoughts are there. Once you let go of them, the negative

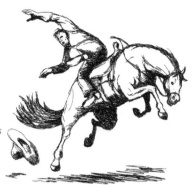

1. *Thoughts are like wild horses. If we lose control, they drag us down to bad moods.*

2. *If we learn how to control them, we can steer our way towards good feelings.*

3. *If we stay present, we will be able to play with our thoughts rather than our thoughts playing with our moods.*

Figure 18.2. Thoughts are like Wild Horses

thoughts, as well as the reality created by them, will instantly vanish into nothingness.

The following real-life example illustrates this point.

A few years ago, when I was going through an extremely stressful situation, I found it hard to stay focused at work. When I tried to stay focused on my job, the thoughts about the problem constantly intruded into my mind to the point that I became very distracted and inefficient. Every day, I went home late. Occasionally I would feel the symptoms of stress—a sense of nausea and discomfort in my stomach, palpitations, and my heart would start to race even while I was just sitting and doing computer work. The constant noise of restless thoughts in my mind was setting off the stress alarm, releasing the stress hormones, leading to all these unpleasant symptoms. All because of a bunch of thoughts! Aargh! Stress is so real when we are in the middle of it!

But once I realized what I was experiencing as stress was nothing but a bunch of stagnated, negative thoughts, I took measures to let go of them and calm myself. I took short five-minute work breaks whenever possible, went to a quiet place, sat still in silence, and practiced some relaxation exercises and calming techniques. I took deep breaths and told myself that everything would be alright if I just let loose those bothersome thoughts. I observed my thoughts as they passively flowed through my mind and tried not to get attached to them. Every now and then, a negative thought entered my mind, but I knew that those negative thoughts created only a momentary, illusory reality. If I didn't pay attention to them, they would have to pass. Unattended guests flee! And so do your negative thoughts! Once they passed, the natural and continuous flow of thoughts resumed and washed away all negativity in my mind. The next good thought waiting in line came forward to serve me. And there you go, I was back to my normal, peaceful, and joyful state of mind.

A Young and Curious Mind

Recently, I was at my uncle's home and his son, my nephew, who is now in college, overheard my conversation with his dad about thoughts and their relation to stress. He was intrigued and inquired, "Is there something called a positive thought and a negative thought? Aren't they all thoughts? How do we differentiate one from another?" I was impressed by his inquisitiveness. There you go! I have a chance to influence a young and curious mind. He got my full attention.

I explained, "Thought is a gift we all are bestowed with at birth. Many thoughts pass through your mind every day. Some of them are good, and some of them are not so good. Positive thoughts are those that are good for you while benefiting others around you, too. At least they should not cause any harm to others. Negative thoughts are those that cause harm to yourself or others. As thoughts pass through your mind, you can pick and choose the thoughts you want. It's like selecting your favorite food at a buffet. There could be one hundred dishes at the buffet, but you don't try to eat them all or you will get indigestion. You just eat in moderation what you like and what is good for your health. That's the secret of keeping a healthy weight. In the same way, *the secret to a healthy mind is choosing only positive thoughts and setting aside negative ones* in the grand buffet of thoughts that pass through your mind."

This explanation and comparison with a buffet seemed to work for him, and he seemed excited about this new idea.

"But what do thoughts have to do with stress?" he asked innocently. As he was eager to learn more, I continued, "Thoughts have everything to do with stress."

"Whenever you get attached to a particular thought and keep incessantly repeating it over in your mind, that's the source of stress."

"It does not matter whether it's a positive or negative thought?" he inquired.

"It does not matter. Thoughts should pass naturally. That's your normal state of mind. Whether you get attached to positive thoughts or negative thoughts, the end result is the same—stress."

"I can understand the bad consequences of getting attached to negative thoughts. But I can't understand what is wrong with an attachment to positive thoughts," he expressed his confusion.

I clarified it for him. "Let's say you went to your favorite restaurant and ordered your favorite food. You felt happy after you had a good portion of the food. What would happen if you continued to eat all day long, sitting there at the restaurant? It would make you sick and you'd throw up. It's your body's way of telling you, 'Hey! Give me some rest.' Even though it's good food, you can't just keep eating nonstop. Similarly, even though it is a positive thought, if you get attached to it and block the thought flow in your mind, it would still cause stress. Getting attached to thoughts, positive or negative, is just an unhealthy state of mind. You don't keep eating incessantly or else your stomach will become over-loaded and your physical health will be adversely affected; *please avoid nonstop thinking or else your mind becomes over-loaded with thoughts and will adversely affect your mental health.* Rest your mind at regular intervals."

"For example, if you keep thinking incessantly about performing well in your basketball game—even though 'performance' is a good thought—you will be so preoc-cupied with it that it may interfere with your natural rhythm of playing the game. You may make more mistakes than usual because *your preoccupied thoughts are interfer-ing with your natural creativity* and the natural flow of your game. You might end up losing the game. That's the reason good coaches emphasize relaxing well before the game. The same holds true for your exams, too! Prepare well for exams but relax well, too."

"Then what should we do?" he asked after carefully lis-tening to all my explaining.

"At best, we should just leave our thoughts alone. Your mind knows best how to use them and rest them.

Thoughts are just neutral entities that we can either use for good or bad. As thoughts pass through your mind, pay attention to the good and helpful ones and use them to accomplish what you have to. And don't think too much about what you should do with your thoughts and how to use them. That in itself is a preoccupation of your mind. As you practice this more, you will understand it more, and you will develop more faith in this simple truth— *nonattachment to thought is a prerequisite for a nonstressed state of mind.* When you are in that state of mind, good things will automatically unfold in your life.

"But, how do we practice nonattachment to thoughts?

"Here is a powerful truth that will help you with that and then I have to take off for the day."

You Are the Power Behind Your Thoughts

You are the creator of your own thoughts; you are the power behind your thoughts. You generate your own unique meaning about everything that you see, hear, taste, touch, and smell through your thoughts. Because you are the power behind your thoughts, you can decide which thoughts to entertain and which to dismiss. *You certainly may not be able to control the first thought that comes to your mind, but you certainly can choose your subsequent thoughts.* You could realize that whatever you are thinking is nothing other than just your thinking—nothing more, nothing less—and when bad thoughts bother you, you don't have to take those thoughts seriously at all. If you turn your back away from them, they will disappear.

Try to apply this next time you face a challenging situation. You will find instant peace of mind. You will no longer react to things unconsciously and stress yourself unnecessarily.

DR. CALM'S PRESCRIPTION

1 ✓ Thoughts are universal phenomena and are the fundamental units of creation. First there is thought and then there is form.

2 ✓ Universal Mind and personal mind are not two separate entities; they are one. Your ego creates a barrier between them. To the extent you are egoistic, that is to that extent you feel separate from the Universal Power. To the extent your ego dissolves, it is to that extent you harness the power of the universe. Calmness dissolves the artificial barrier of ego between the personal and Universal Minds.

3 ✓ Thoughts per se have no animosity toward us. Thoughts are neutral entities. It is we who take those neutral entities and label them good or bad depending on our situations.

4 ✓ If you allow thoughts to flow freely in your mind, you will be naturally happy and cheerful. The moment you obstruct that natural flow, you will start feeling stressful.

5 ✓ Good or positive thoughts are as abundant as bad or negative thoughts. What you reap in your life depends on which thoughts you focus on. Do not encourage negative thoughts or they may become strong negative habits and, once they become strong, it is hard to get rid of them.

6 ✓ Don't try to control thoughts. Control of thoughts is a misnomer. The more you try to control thoughts, the more you will focus on them, making them stronger. You can't control thoughts. You can redirect them. You can choose them. You can steer them in the direction you want.

7 ✓ The very existence of any specific thought depends on your mind's propensity to focus on it. If you don't focus on it, it will go away.

CHAPTER 19

The Inside-Out Nature of Life

*For everything you experience in this world, there will be
a tint of your inner lens on your view of the outer world.*

John was walking down the street and saw a young woman,
Lucy, in her twenties. He thought, *Wow, she is so beautiful.
I should ask her out for a date.*

The person walking next to John is a middle-aged
woman, and she thought, *She looks just like my daughter
who passed away ten years ago in an accident. God bless her
to have a good life.*

The person walking behind John is another young lady, equally beautiful, and she is jealous of Lucy and her beauty. Meanwhile, John's friend comes along and says that Lucy is the meanest girl that he has ever seen. Last night she got into a fight with the bartender and hit him. And she has the most irritating voice you can imagine.

You See this World through an Inner Lens

Do you see how different people looking at the same person have different viewpoints? That means what is external to you doesn't totally determine your experiences. If your experience of life just comes from what is outside of you, then you should experience everything in the world the same way everyone else does. But you don't! You perceive things quite differently even though you are looking at the same object as everyone else. *You see everything through your own unique inner lens that determines your interpretation of what you see in the outside world and thus all your experiences in life.*

Unfortunately, for most people, that inner lens through which they see the world is covered by the dust of restless thoughts, desires, and past experiences that distort their worldview. So, they make wrong assumptions and take wrong actions—which is the source of all the distress they experience.

A Calm Mind Gives You a Distortion-Free View of the World

How do you keep your inner lens clean and clear? The answer is calmness. Yes, calmness is the cleanser of your inner lens. Calmness is what is going to help you achieve a distortion-free, clear view of the world within and around you, thus leading to a clear understanding of life and its myriad processes. You don't realize the true

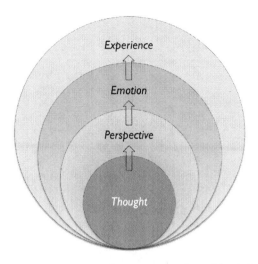

Figure 19.1. Human Experiences Are Created Inside-Out

nature of the world you see unless your mind is devoid of restless thoughts and your inner lens is clean and clear.

You Live in an Inside-Out World *(see Figure 19.1)*

The way you experience the external world is directly related to the world that you are experiencing internally. If you are peaceful within, then everything around you looks calm and serene. If you are happy from within, then you will find happiness everywhere around. However, if you feel irritable within, everything irritates you. If you wear a lens of forgiveness, you will be able to forgive people no matter what. If your mind is prejudiced to begin with, you will judge everything and everyone around you. Notice how your external world is a reflection of your inner world?

I am sure you have met and seen people who fall under all these different categories. *With whom do you want to spend more time? The people who are happy, peaceful, and forgiving, or the people who are upset, irritable, and judgmental?* Whom do you want to be? The former or latter? You can decide for yourself today and start conducting your life that way!

The following real-life example shows how your state of mind influences your perception of the environment and so your experience.

Every year, I take a short vacation far away from professional and family responsibilities. I love to spend time in nature. This time, I was vacationing near a beach. It was evening, around 5 p.m., and I was walking along on this beautiful seashore. I noticed many people enjoying the nice, cool breeze and warm sunlight on a perfect summer day, but I could not derive any happiness from these surroundings. My mind was preoccupied with a problem I was trying to solve in my life. I was quite worried at that time. As much as I tried, I only found myself more restless and uncomfortable.

Finally, I decided to leave the beach and started walking toward the parking lot while thinking, Why can't I enjoy such nice weather on such a beautiful beach on this perfect summer day? Usually, I do.

I decided to drive to my favorite restaurant, hoping that would make me feel a little better. Driving through the city, I was still feeling some sense of discomfort. I reached my favorite restaurant and ordered my favorite food, only it didn't taste right; it didn't taste as good as it usually did. I left more than half my dinner on my plate, uneaten, and with a sense of dissatisfaction, I left the restaurant. Tired and defeated by the restless thoughts in my clouded mind, I drove through the congested, evening traffic to finally reach my hotel room. I retired to bed late that night.

The next day, I woke up feeling refreshed and relaxed after a good night's sleep; I felt much better. I practiced a relaxation exercise and calming technique that helped me regain my peaceful state of mind. That evening, I went to the same beach and I found it pleasant and beautiful. Like everyone around me, I started enjoying the beautiful evening. I walked along the ocean, watching the sunset, observing the waves of the ocean reaching the shore and gracefully being drawn back again into the ocean. An inner calm started pouring out of me, and I felt I was connected to this ocean and to the natural environment around me.

I wondered, "How could I have such a different experience today compared to yesterday on this very same beach? How is that possible?"

Later, I realized that it was my state of mind that determined how I experienced my surroundings. I concluded, "If you are restless from within, even the most beautiful places in the world can't give you happiness and the peace of mind you are looking for. However, if you are calm and relaxed from within, you will find beauty and solace even in the simple things of life. Even simple surroundings will have the most uplifting influence on you."

The moral of this story is that peace of mind and happiness originate from within. In fact, all your experiences are created from within. As you find peace within more and more, you will find that same peace in your external world, too!

What Determines Your Perceptions?

Where do your perceptions come from? Why do you perceive certain things differently than others? There are two things that influence your perceptions: your past conditioning and your state of mind.

Your Past Conditioning

Your past conditioning is the influence of your past experiences on your current perceptions. Sometimes, these influences are so subtle that you are not even aware of them. There might be experiences from your childhood that you don't remember now but that could still be unknowingly and subconsciously influencing your perceptions, emotions, and actions.

Your State of Mind

Another influence on your current perceptions is your current state of mind. You perceive everything in this world through your own unique lens that is built with layers of thoughts and emotions. When your mind is calm, all these layers that cause a distortion of reality dissolve. You see things as they are.

Put Yourself in a Good State of Mind
Before Making Important Decisions

A restless mind distorts the lens through which you see the world. So, *avoid making hasty life decisions when your mind is agitated*, or else you will end up with unnecessary complications. Come what may, make all decisions from a calm state of mind, and you will reap good results.

The following example illustrates how *your emotions and actions are based on your perceptions*—which sometimes can be inaccurate!

As a young man aspiring for a bright career, you recently moved to New York City. It was a chilly Monday morning and the roads are still covered with snow. Wearing a thick winter jacket, you walk toward the subway train station

and you see a woman standing a few feet away on the plat-
form waiting for the train. She is wearing a scarf, and you
can only see her a little bit from the side, but she seems to
be a brilliantly beautiful young woman. Meanwhile, you
hear an announcement that all trains are delayed because
of severe weather conditions. Normally you would have
been frustrated about the delay, but this time you are
quite happy. You think you might chat a little bit with this
beautiful lady, and if things work out, you can invite her
for a cup of coffee. You slowly inch toward her, rehearsing
in your mind how to introduce yourself and start the conversation. As your heart races with excitement, you move
closer to introduce yourself. But, before you can utter your
first words, you have to swallow them back in an awkward
fashion as you can't believe your eyes. As the woman turns
toward you for the first time, you realize that she is not a
young lady as you previously perceived but an old woman
in her seventies. Somehow, you had made a mistake
because of the angle from which you had been looking at
her. How is that possible? Maybe it was the scarf. Maybe
it was the way she was dressed. Thoughts start running
haphazardly in your mind, and the old woman looks at
you, perplexed. You quickly cover up the situation by
saying, "It seems you have been standing here for a while,
and it's quite cold here, and I just wanted to make sure
you were okay. I was sitting on that bench there, and if
you would like to, you can sit there. I am okay standing."
Pleasantly surprised by this random act of kindness, she
smiles back at you and thanks you. Relieved at having
saved face from that awkward experience, you quickly run
out of the subway station and disappear from there.

What if You Perceive the Opposite?

In this example, as our protagonist did, you will have different thoughts about seeing a young woman versus seeing an old woman. If you see an old woman, you might think, "I wonder how her health is. These days, with high health care costs, it's very difficult to pay bills. I hope she has good health insurance. I hope she can afford her medications. Maybe she needs some help?" Conversely, if you see a young woman . . . well, you get the idea.

Do you see how your thought-perceptions shape your reality? Do you see how the reality you perceive triggers certain emotions and actions? Each action leads to certain results, and each result again triggers specific thoughts, and the thought–perception– emotion–action cycle continues (see Figure 19.2).

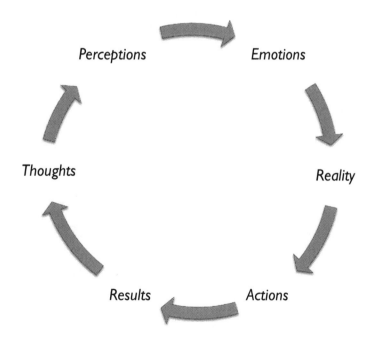

Figure 19.2. The Thought–Perception–Emotion–Action Cycle

Your Perceptions Are Not Always True

Your perceptions are not always true. What appears to be true in one moment could be proven completely wrong in the next moment. You never know! While the previous example was an extreme one, the point is that, we live in our own world shaped by our own perceptions. *Many of our perceptions never get validated.* They mostly remain as assumptions. These assumptions could be false.

Evaluating the Validity of Your Perspectives is the Beginning Point of Change

Self-inquiry is a prerequisite for growth in life. Look at the number of people in certain parts of the world being brought up with hatred toward other nations and religions. They were raised from childhood with the idea that killing others in the name of hatred and religious freedom is okay. Because of this repetitive conditioning since childhood, many have grown into adults harboring hatred in their hearts. The problem is that they haven't stopped for self-assessment and see if their conditioning is harmful or useful. The only true solution to resolve harmful past conditioning is to facilitate a process that helps people look within and see for the first time that the perspectives they were brought up with are just that, their perspectives, and are not necessarily true; they *don't* have to buy into them. They have a choice to entertain alternative perspectives that could lead them to more

> Self-inquiry is a prerequisite for growth in life.

peace, joy, and fulfillment in their lives. That's the beginning point of change. Once people experience it from within, there is no going back.

DR. CALM'S PRESCRIPTION

1 ✓ The reality you perceive is unique to you. You see the world through your own unique lens, and no one else has that lens in this world. Always be aware of this truth.

2 ✓ A restless mind causes distortion of your reality; a calm mind provides a clear perception of your reality. The calmer you are, the closer your perceptions are to reality.

3 ✓ Your world is created inside-out through your thoughts. You not only perceive the world you see but also create the world you perceive.

4 ✓ The world that you are seeing externally is directly related to the world that you are experiencing internally.

5 ✓ Recognize that your perceptions are dependent upon two factors: (1) your state of mind and (2) your past conditioning.

6 ✓ Self-inquiry is a prerequisite for growth in life. Challenge your perceptions every now and then to check whether you hold any false beliefs in your heart or if you are living by truth.

7 ✓ Peace of mind and happiness begin within. If you are not peaceful from within, even the most beautiful places in the world cannot bring you solace. Find inner peace first.

CHAPTER 20

How to Resolve Conflicts and Create Harmony

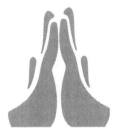

The only true way to harmony and peace in this world is by respecting and understanding the separate realities we live in.

Conflict Means a Difference in Viewpoints (see Figure 20.1)

If you're like most people, you get into arguments with your friends, colleagues, or family members because of a difference in viewpoints, not because you hate each other. But eventually, these differences in opinion might lead to hatred. You both find it difficult to let go of these thought-perceptual differences in your

213

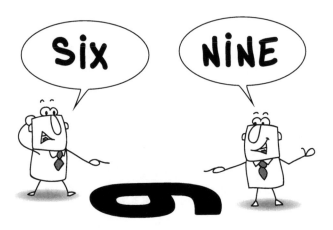

Figure 20.1. Difference in Perspectives

personal minds. Although these conflicts may have happened in the past and are now nothing but pure memories, your attachment to those thought-memories perpetuate the negative feelings and the conflict in your current relationship. If you could learn to let go of those hurtful thoughts and memories, you could reestablish that good relationship you once had.

Do Not Become Defiant When Your Reality Is Challenged

When we are challenged by situations or people with different perceptions, we feel defiant and sharply disagree with them. But we can avoid this defiance by ridding ourselves of the perception that our relative reality is the *only* reality. When you wake up to that fact—that what you have been thinking as real your entire life is just your own perception, and at times it could be totally wrong—your defiance will dissolve and will be replaced by true understanding.

If you understand the possibility of separate and personalized realities, you will not become defiant, and thus avoid conflict. You will simply see it as another perspective that is very real for the other person. You become more understanding of the people around you. You stop imposing your perspectives on others. The people around you will love you because you understand them so well. They will find it easy to relate to you.

He Who Understands Others Conquers the World

Understanding others and getting along with people is the key to success in this world. Along with competence in your field, your relationships with others are pivotal for success. Poor relationships hinder success and are often the limiting factor for many, even for people who are very knowledgeable in their field. Practicing how to understand and establish rapport with others will help you conquer even the toughest challenges.

> Understanding others and getting along with people is the key to success in this world.

The World of Relative Realities

Let's do a small activity together. Close your eyes for a moment. Count back from 25 to 1 slowly and steadily. Now relax and take a deep breath. Think about 10 absolute realities you know. An *absolute reality* is something that all people in the world agree and acknowledge to be absolutely true. Now, open your eyes and write them down on a piece of paper. If you are able to list 10 absolute realities, think of 10 more and write them down, too. After you finish writing down 20, then write down as many more that you can possibly think of.

A few examples of absolute realities are:

1. Earth is round and revolves around the Sun.
2. The Sun rises in the east.
3. The oceans are made of water.
4. Objects thrown into the air fall because of gravity.

A few examples of *relative realities* are:

1. The iPhone is the best phone in the world. (Maybe it is for some people, but not for everyone.)
2. The United States is the richest and the most powerful nation in the world. (Not anymore and not according to everyone.)
3. My religion is the greatest. (That may be true for you, but not for everyone.)
4. All homes are made of wood. (Not really; there are homes made of glass and concrete, too.)

When you finish this exercise, put aside the pen and paper and take a moment to reflect on how many absolute realities you came up with. Maybe it was 10, or maybe 20, or maybe a few more. Most people can barely come up with a list of 10 absolute realities and a majority of them are related to Earth and our solar system, which are absolute physical realities. That's it. The rest are just relative realities, depending on how you think about them. Relative realities are limitless. Now, think about all the 7.4 billion people in this world, all of whom think about everything around them the way they want to. Do you see that there are infinite, separate realities in this world?

Do you immediately see why there is so much conflict throughout the world? Do you see why it's hard for people to agree on certain things, even in the closest relationships like husband and wife, parents and children, or brothers and sisters? The only true way to harmony and peace in this world is to respect the separate realities we all live in. *Where you can understand others' perspectives, do so; if you can't, simply agree to disagree. If everyone does this, most of the problems in this world will be solved quickly.*

Seeing the Absolute Reality

This is one world. Yet each one of us live in our unique personal world, the product of our mental constructs. What a paradox!

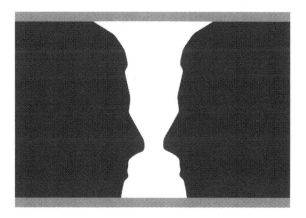

Figure 20.2. Optical Illusion

Even though there is One Absolute Reality, each of us live in our own personal reality shaped by our own thoughts. *We are deeply engrossed in it, truly take it to our heart, and act accordingly all our life,* without considering that other people can see the same world very differently. Figure 20.2 and the explanation below demonstrate this point.

There are two *relative* realities in this picture: the *flower vase* and the *two people looking at each other.* But either reality is just your perception, your own relative reality, which you believe to be the only reality until you see both realities in the picture. To take this a step further, beyond those two relative realities there is one absolute reality—*black and white lines on a dark background.* The same way, *in life there are multiple relative realities in any given situation, but there is One Absolute Reality.* And that Absolute Reality will be apparent to you when your mind is absolutely calm, without even a single flicker of restless thought.

Look Out for A-ha! Experiences

Each time you experience this Truth, you will have a profound A-ha! experience—the realization that helps you see the ephemeral nature of relative perceptions and the Absolute Reality behind every situation. That new understanding opens up a new world and a new way to experience life. Life is nothing but a series of such realizations that help you learn, grow, and slowly inch toward perfection. So, keep looking for A-ha! moments. Each such profound realization takes you to a higher level of understanding.

There is More Excitement and Joy in Life with Higher Understanding

Life is like climbing Mount Everest. Every 100 feet, you have a new vista opening up what you could not see when you were down below. When you finally reach the peak of the mountain, your view and understanding of the ground and life below is limitless. You can see everything around you with great clarity and detail at a level that you could not see when you were down at the base of the mountain. There is more excitement and joy at the peak than when you were at the base of the mountain. So, do not settle for less. Aim for higher understanding in life. With better understanding comes better life, more happiness and success. Isn't that the goal of life?

> Aim for higher understanding in life. With better understanding comes better life.

Redefining Your Perspective

Many people live in their limited perspectives all their lives. For example, if you think that you can never succeed, you will continually fail in life. If you think that you will never make enough money, you will be poor. If you think that you never have enough time, you will always be in a time crunch. You see, *you are a prisoner of your own thoughts.* You obstruct your innate potential by constantly imposing limiting thoughts on yourself. And sometimes we live in someone else's perspectives. We let others' opinions limit us.

When your mind is calm, you see things for what they are. You will clearly see your true potential and not be bound by the limiting perceptions you or others may have about you, allowing your innate talent to flow unhindered. This is the key to success!

Going Beyond Limited Perspectives

The great thinkers of the world are ahead of their time because they could see what was not obvious to most others. For example, many decades ago, everyone used to believe that stomach ulcers were caused by spicy foods. In 1982, Dr. Robin Warren and Dr. Barry Marshall proposed that a bacterium called *Helicobacter pylori* causes stomach ulcers. Immediately, they were ridiculed by the establishment scientists and doctors who did not believe that any bacteria could live in the acidic environment of the stomach. It took years before the scientific community saw the evidence and accepted this hypothesis. Two decades later, in 2005, both doctors were recognized for their life-changing work with the Nobel Prize. So, *step out of your comfort zone and dare to think outside the box!*

Resolving Conflicts

Do you know the reason for the high rate of divorce and relationship failure in current society? It's because of conflicts stemming from false assumptions and misunderstandings. For example, if your spouse assumes that you did something wrong and keeps blaming you without ever asking for your perspective on that situation, how would that make you feel?

The following example illustrates how false assumptions can create conflict in a marriage.

Once, a wise man noticed a husband and wife loudly arguing right outside their home. The wife angrily said something and forcefully went inside their home. The wise man inquired, "What happened?" The husband said, "We were just cleaning our home and disposing of all unnecessary objects. There is so much garbage that my wife packed everything in at least a dozen trash bags. I was ready to carry them to the dumpster. I parked my wife's car in front of our house, went inside, and carried a few trash bags outside and placed them in the trunk of the car. The next thing that happened was that my wife came out of the house, saw what I was doing, became very upset, said a few nasty things to me, and angrily went back inside."

"Why?" the wise man asked. The husband replied, "I don't know why. She didn't tell me the reason." The husband continued, "I think she was upset because she felt that I was using her car to carry all that trash instead of mine. I couldn't believe she was thinking so selfishly when I have been helping her clean up the house and carrying all the trash out. Even though I have a thousand other things to do, I have set aside time specifically to help her out, and this is the thanks I get in return," the husband retorted painfully.

"Did you confirm with her that's the actual reason for her being upset or are you just assuming it?" the wise man inquired. "Well, she said the car was going to get dirty this way! So, I assume she doesn't want me to use her car. So selfish! So I said a few bad things back in response to her upset behavior," the husband burst out. After thoughtfully considering what happened, the wise man advised, "Why don't you confirm your assumptions? If you find out what you assumed to be true, then I won't stop you if you still want to be upset with her." After he said that, the wise man retired for that evening.

The next day, when the wise man went on his evening walk, the husband hastily approached him with excitement to tell him what happened the previous night. When he asked his wife why she was upset, she replied, "I asked you not to carry so many trash bags at once in the car. But, you didn't do as asked." The man had replied, "What's the big deal? We have so many trash bags and I thought it would take fewer trips to the dumpster if I could squeeze more of them together at once. I thought I was being very efficient."

The wife had replied, "But, I didn't want you to squeeze them all together. Some of the bags have liquid materials inside. If you squeeze them, they are going to leak in the car! I told you that!" The man replied, "No! You never told me." "Yes, I did," the wife responded quickly. "You were right there when I was mentioning it to you; you were just pulling up the car in front of the house."

The husband responded, "Whatever you said I couldn't hear because you were shouting from inside the house and I was outside getting the car ready and the car engine was on. I didn't even know that you were trying to tell me something." The wife looked at him incredulously and said, "I thought all this time you were just ignoring me and being disrespectful despite my pleas to be careful that the trash bags might leak. I thought you were just being stubborn and didn't want to listen to me, even it is for your own good."

The husband replied, "Huh! Do you see now that I was

not being stubborn or disrespectful? You see . . . I am not a bad guy." For the first time, the wife saw the situation from a new perspective and understood his side of the story. The husband also realized his wife's point of view and his anger toward her disappeared. With that, the tension in the relationship dissolved instantly.

Negative Assumptions Can Destroy Even the Strongest Relationships

In this example, do you see how false assumptions and alternative viewpoints created conflict? Most quarrels start with petty arguments like this. Eventually, people start fighting badly, straining their relationships and becoming hostile toward each other. If not for the wise man's counsel to clarify the assumptions, the true reason for their upset feelings would have been buried forever.

The Mantra for Successful Relationships

Avoid assumptions, clarify when needed, and always try to understand. Without true understanding, love cannot flourish, and human relationships perish. True understanding comes from being curious about other people's perspectives without being judgmental. *When understanding is established between two hearts, even the most difficult conflicts dissolve instantly and upset feelings are replaced by feelings of love and kindness.*

DR. CALM'S PRESCRIPTION

1 Most conflicts in this world are because of a difference in viewpoints and not because people hate each other. But if the differences are not solved quickly, they can turn into hatred.

2 People are often deeply stuck in their own perspectives, and sometimes they are not even aware of it. This "stuck" position becomes a limiting factor in their growth and success both personally and professionally. Don't be stuck! Try alternate perspectives.

3 The next time you feel you have been treated unfairly, see whether it's just your perspective or the truth. If you think it might be just your perspective, try to know the truth. This will save you a lot of misery down the road.

4 Most people are prisoners of their thoughts and struggle to free themselves from that prison. Practicing calmness helps you dissolve the prison walls of limiting thoughts.

5 Know that there are few absolute realities and infinite separate realities. Whatever you perceive is your own truth, others may or may not share your opinion. They have that right.

6 When your reality is challenged, don't get defiant but be curious and look for an A-ha! moment behind it. If you do that consistently, you will expand your perspective and reap good results in life.

7 Understanding and getting along with people is the key to success in this world. A mantra for productive relationships is: avoid assumptions, clarify when needed, and always try to understand.

CHAPTER 21

How to Overcome Mood Swings

Moodiness is a dangerous illness. The cure to moodiness is daily practice of even-mindedness.

Moods—The Greatest Enemy to Your Relationships

So many people in this world are victims of mood swings. One moment they are fine, and the next moment, heaven only knows why, they turn moody. Moodiness is not a good trait. It makes you quite unpredictable, and people around you might start avoiding you if you are always moody. By being moody and

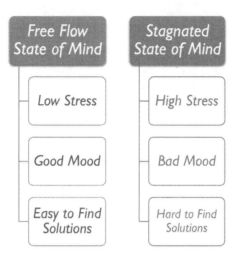

Figure 21.1. Good Mood vs. Bad Mood

irritable, you not only create misery for yourself but also for your family and friends. Just because people continue to tolerate you and your moods, it does not give you permission to continue to be temperamental. *One day, even the most patient and kindhearted person who has silently tolerated your moods for years might leave you because, chronic bad temper can erode other people's good feelings for you.* This is especially true in a close relationship like marriage where one person's moods and behavior strongly affect the partner. So, get a handle on your emotions. Stop being moody!

The Real Reason Behind Moodiness

People often wonder what makes them moody. The answer? *It is your bad habits of thinking that solidify into moodiness.* Knowingly or unknowingly, some people carry these tendencies from childhood, and over time, they turn into strong habits. Children might learn these traits from their parents and other adults they observe. If children are not taught how to correctly handle their emotions and moods, they develop maladaptive behaviors. It is important to teach children how their thoughts drive their emotions and moods, and how to choose good thoughts and good mood.

Good Moods vs. Bad Moods (see Figure 21.1)

In your mind, thoughts flow freely. As long as you let them flow freely, you remain happy and peaceful. That is a good mood. The moment you block the flow of thoughts in your mind by attaching to thoughts, you impede their natural flow and you feel unhappy and distressed. That's a bad mood. We often get attached to past negative experiences or an imagined, fearful future. Persistent focus on negative thoughts leads to a bad mood. The way to bounce back to a good mood is to allow thoughts to pass freely in your mind. You can do this by practicing *thought detachment*. Realize that it doesn't matter what kind of thoughts you have in your mind. Whether good thoughts, bad thoughts, worried thoughts, negative thoughts, positive thoughts, or some other thoughts, they are just thoughts. They are supposed to flow freely and vanish into nothingness. If you allow them to pass, they will pass. If you hold onto them, they will stay.

Why Do People Overreact?

Some people overreact to every little thing. That's because they are in a bad mood. *Moods determine your response to stressors.* Is there a day in your life when you were so stressed and irritated? Either because your boss reprimanded you, you have a big bill to pay shortly, may be your kid is sick at home, or because of something else, you are so stressed that everything around you starts to annoy you. Even innocuous sounds can elicit a bad response from you—the ringing phone, the chiming text message, the swooshing e-mail—everything becomes a source of irritation. However, the truth is that they are not to blame. It's *your own bad mood that attracts like a magnet the sharp nails of stressors that turn your day into a painful series of adverse events.*

The Emotional Sore Spots

Sometimes, we are emotionally sensitive and overreact in a similar way to being physically sore and sensitive, as illustrated by the following real-life example. One of my friends related this story to me.

A few years ago, I had some back pain and went for physical therapy. When the therapist started applying pressure to my back, there were certain places on my back that were very painful, and some places that were not. Wincing in pain, I retorted, "Why do you apply so much pressure on certain parts and less pressure on others? It's really painful."

The therapist courteously replied, "Sir! I have been applying the same pressure all over your back, but it seems that there are certain sore spots on your back that are causing pain even with minimal pressure."

I thought, "All this time I am blaming the therapist for applying too much pressure, but in fact, it's my internal sore spots that are causing the pain and not the external pressure being applied."

Isn't it the same way with regard to our emotional reactivity? There are people who are emotionally sensitive, and it does not take much to elicit a bad response from them. It seems that they have emotional sore spots in their minds that can be triggered even by minor pressures of life.

A Good Mood Is a Cushion of Invincibility

However, *when you are in a good mood, you develop a cushion of protection around you, and the nails of stressors cannot penetrate*

Low/Bad Mood	High Stress	Not Able to See Solutions
High/Good Mood	Low Stress	Able to See Solutions Easily

Figure 21.2. Relationships Between Mood, Stress, and Problem-Solving Ability

your happy state of mind. When you are in a good mood, even bad incidents do not bother you. You take them in stride and move on. You easily see solutions and effortlessly overcome problems. You finish the tasks at hand efficiently and have more time to enjoy your life. Moreover, when you are emotionally strong, you remain poised even under pressure. You stand unshaken even in the midst of worlds falling apart. *You remain calm in the midst of chaos.*

A Good Mood and Stress Can't Live Together

If you try to keep yourself in a good mood, stress walks out of your life. A good mood and stress can't live together. *Fake it until you make it!* Don't let your inner distress overflow to the outside. Keep smiling and be composed. I am not advising you not to address the challenges you face, but keep calm and don't yield to moods, even under pressure. With practice, you can win over your moods. Eventually, you will be transformed from a moody person into an emotionally stable person.

> Don't let your inner distress overflow to the outside. Keep smiling and be composed.

How to Put Yourself in a Good Mood

There are three simple ways to put yourself in a good mood:

1. **Let your thoughts flow freely.** That's the natural state of your mind. As long as you do not obstruct the flow of thoughts, you will be in good mood.

2. **Do not pay attention to negative thoughts,** even though you may feel compelled to do so. If you already find yourself in a bad mood because you focused on negative thoughts, turn your attention away from them. Just do not yield to them. The moment you decide to let the negative thoughts pass, the natural flow of positive thoughts will wash them away and you will find yourself in a good mood again.

3. **Focus on happy thoughts.** Whatever thoughts you choose to focus on become your moods. Focus on happy thoughts and you will find yourself in a happy mood. Focus on sad thoughts and I guarantee that you will find yourself in a bad mood. Know that it is within your power to choose the thoughts you want to focus on and so the resulting feelings. Even when you are facing difficult circumstances, see beyond them and focus on something positive. The undeniable truth of life is that even in situations that appear hopeless, a ray of hope exists and awaits you. If necessary, create happy thoughts. That's totally under your control!

Be the Hero of Your Life

Even-mindedness is the solution to moodiness. If you keep smiling inwardly and maintain an attitude of even-mindedness at all times, external circumstances will affect you less. Your own internal world will rule your life. Anyone can smile when things are going well in their life. But only a hero can smile even when things are not going well. A hero knows *every difficulty in life is a temporary phase, and sooner or later, that tough phase must pass, and a good phase must arrive.* A hero knows that's the nature of life. Decide today that is the way you want to live the rest of your life. *Be the hero of your life!*

DR. CALM'S PRESCRIPTION

1. Moodiness results in unpredictable emotions and reactions, thus making it very difficult for people to understand and get along with you. They will live in a constant state of doubt and fear not knowing what will set your mood off in the wrong direction.

2. No one likes to stay around moody people, especially in close relationships. Your moodiness can adversely affect the relationship. Take control of your moods today before it is too late.

3. Moodiness results from bad habits of thinking that get solidified into moods over time. The seeds for moodiness are often sowed in your childhood. But you can undo them by conscious choice.

4. By developing the habit of calmness and learning to put yourself in a good mood at will, you become invincible to mood swings.

5. Next time, when a negative mood approaches you, watch and laugh at it. Tell the mood that you are awake. You are present. In that state of wakefulness, moods cannot bother you. As you practice this daily, eventually all the bad moods relinquish their grip on you.

6. It is essential to put yourself in a good mood consistently for maximal success in life. When you are in a good mood, it is much easier to find solutions to your problems and accomplish the tasks at hand.

7. The secret to putting yourself in a good mood is to (1) let your thoughts flow freely in your mind, (2) not focus on negative thoughts, and (3) direct your mind to think positive thoughts.

CHAPTER 22

How to Develop Even-Mindedness

If you are waiting for everything in your life to be perfect before you can be happy, you are sure to be disappointed.

Life Bears You No Animosity, It Is Just a Roller-Coaster Ride

What is even-mindedness? Even-mindedness is a state of mind where you are not swayed either by good or bad news. You take both equally. You are calm no matter what. You do not get ruffled by life situations. *Even-mindedness starts with realizing that life is neutral; life bears you no animosity.* Life is just a roller-coaster ride that takes you up and down during

233

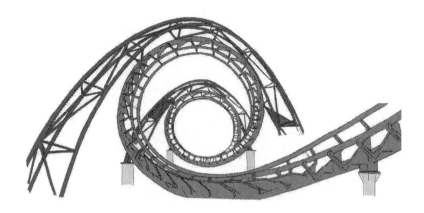

Figure 22.1. Ups and Downs in Life Are Normal, Like a Roller Coaster Ride

your journey (see figure 22.1). The ups and downs are inevitable. Then why don't you stop complaining and start enjoying the ride? Once you accept the inevitability of the ups and downs in life, the ride becomes more relaxing and enjoyable. Getting scared of this journey and jumping off the roller-coaster is not going to help you. It's only going to hurt you more.

Some people are always on an emotional roller-coaster, going from too much excitement to too much disappointment. They live like that forever without realizing that it is their habitual thinking that is switching the roller-coaster of their emotions off and on. It is emotionally draining to live like that. So, *try to develop even-mindedness and you will feel much more peaceful.*

Keep Saying, "I Don't Mind"

When good things happen in life, enjoy them. When things don't happen as expected, gracefully accept them. Do not label them as bad and sinister. When you develop an attitude of even-mindedness, the roller-coaster journey of life becomes easier to ride. Life becomes neutral to you. It becomes your friend. People around you become more welcoming, helpful, and seek your company. They will equally enjoy the ride with you as you help them see this truth.

Restlessness Results in a Fragmented World View

Realize that, at the core of our being, we all are the same undivided, pure consciousness. Imagine you are seeing the image of the moon in a mirror. That unbroken mirror can be compared to your pure, undivided consciousness. Let us say someone throws a stone at the mirror and it breaks into pieces. You look down to pick up the mirror, and instead of seeing one moon, you see multiple moons in multiple pieces of mirror. And the moon appears to be fragmented. Even though there is just one moon, why do you see so many, and why does the moon appear to be fragmented? It is because the mirror in which you're viewing the moon is fragmented. In the same way, restlessness is the stone that fragments our consciousness so we see a fragmented view of the world, creating an illusion of multiple realities.

Calmness Brings Wholeness to Your Life

Calmness is the glue that mends the broken mirror of consciousness and makes it whole again. With that, the illusion of separate realities dissolves, and your consciousness beholds one complete reality. *To reclaim the lost purity and wholeness of your consciousness is the highest purpose of life.* When you reach that state, nothing bothers you because you stop seeing things as incomplete. You see everything as complete. You stand above the dualities of this world. Even the things that trouble most people will not bother you because you don't see them as negative but as the other side of the same positive situation. In fact, the concept of negative and positive disappears, and the concept of completeness enters in its stead.

How to Rise Above Dualities

Look at the circle in the Figure 22.1. If you divide this circle and only see half of it at once (see Figures 22.2 and 22.3), you obviously think that there are two semicircles, one above and one below. You might label the semicircle above "positive" and the semicircle below "negative." But when both parts are combined to form one complete circle, the differences and dualities vanish. You just see one continuum that has neither beginning nor end; it's just one circle. The same way, when you perceive the wholeness of the world, you automatically lose the tendency to see things as good and bad, positive and negative, superior and inferior. You start looking at everything with even-mindedness. It's like looking at the complete circle for the first time (see Figure 22.4). And when you do that, life's challenges bother you less. You know it is all one circle of life, and it is inevitable to have ups and downs. You know that these positives and negatives (dualities of life) exist because of the relative realities created by your restless thoughts. That understanding is liberating!

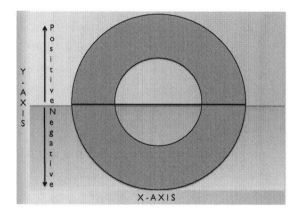

Figure 22.1. You see both positive and negative aspects but still perceive them as two separate entities, not one whole entity.

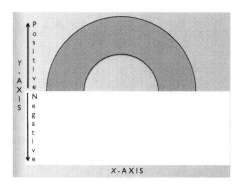

Figure 22.2. You see only the positive aspect here.

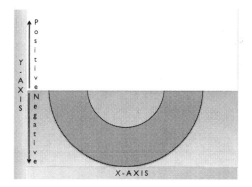

Figure 22.3. You see only the negative aspect here.

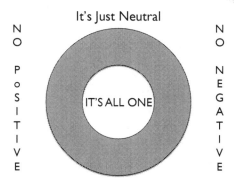

Figure 22.4. It's Just Neutral. You see neither the negative
or positive aspect. You rise above dualities.

DR. CALM'S PRESCRIPTION

1 ✓ Even-mindedness means you do not mind whether you receive good news or bad news; you are calm no matter what. It means being unruffled no matter what your life situation is.

2 ✓ Know that life has no animosity toward you. In life, everything happens for a reason. You may not know the reason today, but it is for your highest good. If you keep this perspective and are accepting of life as it is, you will remain even-minded.

3 ✓ When your expectations are not met, instead of getting upset, practice saying, "I don't mind." That is a good way to remain neutral to life's situations.

4 ✓ When something good happens in life, enjoy it. Don't get too excited, though. The next downturn is around the corner. That's the nature of life—it's a roller-coaster ride. If you are prepared for that ride and are expecting a downturn, it is less likely that you will be taken aback when bad things happen.

5 ✓ Duality—pain and pleasure, light and darkness, up and down, good and bad, cold and hot—is an inherent part of the nature of this Creation. Realizing this truth simplifies life.

6 ✓ When you see the oneness behind all duality, you will see the neutrality of this Creation.

7 ✓ Restlessness results in fragmented view of this world. Calmness brings wholeness to life and helps you rise above the duality of this Creation. Practice calmness.

CHAPTER 23

How to Overcome Karma

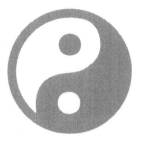

The deeper your presence, the higher your awareness and the lesser your karma. *

Awareness, Experience, and Subconscious Memory

Two things are needed to experience life: first, thoughts themselves, and second, awareness of your thoughts. During wakeful periods when you are aware of thoughts, you experience life. When you are deeply asleep, your awareness levels drop,

---

* Definition: Karma is the sum of all the good and bad that you have done in the past, whether knowingly or unknowingly. These past actions, thoughts, and memories are an integral part of your subconscious mind and could determine your future thoughts and actions.

239

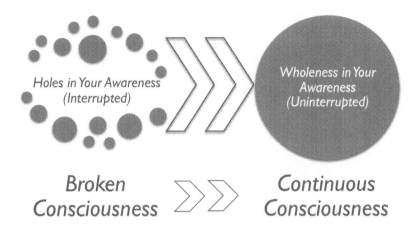

Figure 23.1. Broken Consciousness vs. Continuous Consciousness

and thus you do not remember anything that happens during that time. Without awareness, there is no memory of your experience.

Your past experiences and the dreams are stored in your subconscious mind, whether you remember them or not. Those subconscious memories continue to influence your life whether you are aware of them or not. That's the reason sometimes you (re)act unreasonably and rather unpredictably; it's as if you are driven by an invisible force to behave that way. That invisible force is your subconscious influence, also known as *invisible habits*. As your awareness levels rise, the subconscious influences fade. Their grip loosens and you will be able to act out of free choice rather than by the compulsion of invisible habits.

Broken Awareness Is a Low State of Awareness

Most of us live in the past or future, stepping out of the present moment—a state of broken awareness (see Figure 23.1). That's a low state of awareness. The more you live in the present, the higher your state of awareness. In that state, no restless thought can pass your mind without your notice. You are like a highly vigilant police officer who at once quickly spots the mischievous thief. *When you make it a habit to stay present, the thieves of restless thoughts cannot steal your happiness.*

Awareness is not a magical or mystical word. It simply means being aware of what is happening within and around you. If you are not aware that the stress in your life is a result of thought attachment and stagnation, then all the zillion measures you take to be stress-free yield only transient relief. You might go for a walk, exercise, listen to music, participate in sports, read a book, drink, smoke, use drugs, or do any other activity, but they will only bring temporary stress relief. But if you address the root cause of stress, which is thought attachment, you can have lasting results.

When you make it a habit to stay present, the thieves of restless thoughts cannot steal your happiness.

The Liberating Truth about Your Destiny

Your problems are not in control of your destiny—you are! *No matter what your situation is or what kind of problems you face, they can't exist without you thinking about them.* This truth is liberating! You suddenly break free of all the limitations in your mind. You feel joyful, peaceful, and content, despite unchanged external circumstances. That's a wonderful state to live in. Once you live in that pure state of mind, you will never want to come back to an ordinary, restless state of mind. This happened to me when I was first exposed to the Three Principles. All the restless thoughts vanished from my mind as if someone vacuumed them out.

When you fall down from that peak state of mind, and if you are aware of your descent, you can quickly regain it. With practice, you can remain there longer and longer. You can go about all the activities in your life without slipping to a lower state of mind. If you do slip, it will be transient. In this process, you automatically attain sustained states of higher awareness.

Living in the Present Eliminates Stress

Being in the present moment is not a miraculous feat. It is simple, and you get better with practice. First, understand that *being present is your natural state of mind.*

Second, know that you are already there. *Know that there is only one moment—this moment.* Whatever happened a moment ago is no longer present. It has already passed. And the next moment has not come yet. The future is not yet here. So, you are always in the present, whether you are ware of it or not.

Third, to more fully live in the present *simply "go with the flow."* When you go with the flow, your mind does not dwell on the past nor is it anxious about the future. It just takes whatever thought comes in and is present with it completely. The longer you practice this, the more fully and completely present you will become.

Imagine you are a traveler who has lost the way; you are tired and looking for a place to rest and refresh. In your search, you find a valley of peace to your right. You notice some stairs leading down into the valley, and you start walking down them. The more time you spend walking down the stairs, the deeper you go into the valley. The deeper you descend into the valley, the more peaceful and refreshed you feel. In the same way, the more time you stay present, the deeper the sense of peace you feel. The longer you stay there, the longer you want to stay there.

The more you are anchored to the present, the harder it is for the ferocious waves of restless thoughts to disturb and pull you out of your peaceful haven. It's like being at the bottom step in the valley of peace; it is much more difficult to leave the valley if you are on the bottom step rather than the top step.

When you are present, stress must be absent

When you are present, stress must be absent. Neither the dark memories of the past nor the insecure imaginations of the future can penetrate the infallible walls of your intensely present state of mind. Your mind becomes a safe and dependable refuge that harbors only the thoughts of the moment. *As you dwell in the present longer and longer, experiencing deeper and greater peace, the bad experiences of the past will be erased, and the fearful thoughts of the future will vanish.* With that, karma will flee!

The Invisible Force that Drives Your Destiny

Much of your life is governed by your subconscious memory. How often do you get up in the morning and start looking at Google maps for the location of your office? Do you use a GPS every day to go to work? Well, if you're like most people, you probably don't. Why? That's because subconsciously, you already know your way to work and how to get back home. You probably don't even pay that much attention to the road you drive to work and home. Many times, you are not even aware that you are taking the right exit to get home. It just automatically happens, even when you are listening to music or not particularly paying attention.

Imagine if you got up every day and had forgotten how to drive back and forth to work and home, and you had to think about every turn to take. You would go mad! Without subconscious memory borne out of habit, you couldn't easily perform any tasks in your life. Those subconscious influences allow you to do things even when you are not consciously aware of your actions—like driving to and from work every day. Some of these subconscious influences on your life are good, but some are not so good.

You Don't Have to Be a Prisoner of Your Subconscious Habits

Knowingly or unknowingly, whatever you did in the past influences your present and shapes your future. You can call it *karma*. But know that karma loses its grip if you are highly conscious— being totally present and aware of what's happening around you. That gives you a great deal of control over your destiny despite subconscious, karmic influences. In that highly conscious state, your ability to exercise your free choice increases dramatically. You could use your willpower and follow the dictates of wisdom rather than being the slave of unwanted, subconscious habits. Thus, you break free from your past actions, subconscious influences, and bad habits and so from the prison of karma.

The Greater Your Awareness, the Less Your Karma Affects You

Understand that the law of cause and effect is nothing but karma. As long as you are in the state of broken consciousness, for every action there is an equal and opposite reaction. So, whether you want to or not, you will have to endure the consequences of the good and bad actions you performed in the past, unless you rise to the state of unbroken awareness/continuous consciousness. The higher your state of consciousness, the less influence karma has on you.

> The higher your state of consciousness, the less influence karma has on you.

Attaining unbroken awareness (continuous consciousness) is the highest purpose of life. When a person reaches that state, he or she has risen above all the limitations imposed by habits and subconscious influences and will be liberated from the iron jaws of time—the past, present, or future.

DR. CALM'S PRESCRIPTION

1 For you to experience life, two things are needed: first, thoughts themselves, and second, awareness of your thoughts.

2 If you are like most people, you are restless and are at a low state of awareness, and you think that is normal. But when you experience deep calmness and higher states of awareness, you will realize this is your normal and better self.

3 Being "highly aware" means being totally absorbed in the present moment and being aware of it.

4 Being in the present moment means being totally with your present thoughts and not being drifted away to the past or future. Practice being in the moment.

5 Know that karma is the sum of all the good and bad that you have done in the past, whether knowingly or unknowingly. These past actions, thoughts, and memories are an integral part of your subconscious mind and could determine your future thoughts and actions.

6 When you reach higher states of awareness, karma loses its grip, and you will no longer be compelled by your past. You can consciously choose your present thoughts and actions, setting a new direction in life.

7 Attaining a state of unbroken awareness or continuous consciousness is the highest purpose of life. In that state, you will remain ever peaceful, joyful, and content.

CHAPTER 24

Defy the Gravity of Your Past and Create a Promising Future

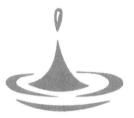

Past is a memory. Future is an imagination. Present is the place everything happens. So stay present.

The Past: A Journey into Your Memory

A couple went to a psychotherapist for marriage counseling. The therapist asked the wife to explain the events that led them to the breaking point of their marriage. The wife recounted all the terrible things her husband had done to her (according to her point of view) and started crying. Then the husband detailed all the horrendous deeds of his wife (according to his point of view) and became distraught. The session ended with the couple feeling more upset with each other than ever.

They went home wondering why they were feeling even more dejected after the session. Isn't it supposed to help? They justified themselves by thinking, "Well, it's unrealistic to expect results after just one session." So, they went back to the therapist again and again, only to discover that their relationship was getting worse and worse. They spent a lot of money, and the little good that remained in their relationship seemed to be slipping way. Their relationship was now teetering dangerously on a precipice, and they were on the verge of separation and divorce. They were confused and didn't know what to do next. But, even in the midst of all this confusion and misery, one thing they were sure of—they were not going back to the therapist*; it was not helping at all.

---

* This is not to bash anyone. There are many wonderful psychotherapists helping thousands of people every day and I have great respect for them. This is rather a real-life example where it demonstrates a specific point that dwelling and digging into your ugly past can be harmful.

Do Not Dig into the Ugly Feelings of Your Past

Do you know why they felt more miserable after going to therapy? Why do some people spend years in therapy without much improvement? It's because some therapists (not all) make you recite all the bad experiences of the past, and as you dig out those ugly thoughts, the negative feelings that were buried deep down

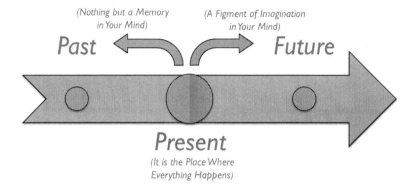

Figure 24.1. The Past and the Future Exist in the Present

resurface. Sometimes, people dig up events that happened years ago. The more you do this, the worse you feel. That is what happened to the couple who went to therapy in our example. As they focused on negative feelings, they couldn't help but feel unhappy. *You become whatever you focus on. You feel whatever you focus on.*

The Past Has No Life in and of Itself

People often get caught up in thoughts of the past as if brooding over their dark past helps create a brighter future; instead, they reap stress. Focusing on adverse events of your past creates negative feelings that make you miserable. *Past has no life in and of itself unless you breathe life into it by thinking about it and bringing it back to the present.* Do not pay attention to the negative events of your past no matter how dark they were. Just learn from your past and move on. The only function of the past is to serve as teacher.

What happened a year ago, a month ago, a day ago, or even a minute ago has already passed. That's why it is called the *past; it already happened*, and there is nothing you can do about it. However, your memory of what happened a minute ago is fresher than your memory of what happened a year ago, making it seem it is still present. But things that happened a minute ago are as unalterable as things that happened years ago.

Breaking Free of the Limitations of the Past

Because of this wonderful gift we have called *memory*, we remember the past. Imagine if you couldn't remember anything more than what happened in your life in the last minute. What happens then? Well, you live moment to moment. You no longer have the opportunity to misuse your mind to brood over the past. You don't remember who yelled at you five minutes ago, how mean your boss was to you yesterday, how emotionally traumatized you were by the war you went through ten years ago, nor who abused you as a child twenty years ago. Nothing; you remember nothing. You are *free* from the horrible memories and limitations of the past! You just live moment to moment.

But, what happens if you have no memory? "Oh! I can't imagine such a situation . . . what happens to me if I become like that?" If you can't remember anything that happened more than a minute ago, do you realize how chaotic your life would be? Imagine you went to sleep last night perfectly fine, but by the time you woke up in the morning, all your memories were erased. You can't remember who you are. You don't remember that you have to brush your teeth, take a shower, eat breakfast, drive to work—nothing. Moving forward, you can't form any habits. Everything you do, you forget within a minute. Thank God we are not like that. Our lives would be purely at the mercy of fate.

Memory Is a Gift—Use It Wisely

I have used this extreme example to show you how vital memory is for your survival and progress in life. Memory is a practical tool to remember those things that you want to—like mistakes, for instance—but that you do not want to repeat again. Memory is a tool that builds habits in your life, sometimes consciously and sometimes subconsciously. That's all. Memory is just a practical tool. Once you are done using this tool, put it away.

If you decide not to think about it, the hurt from the past loses its grip on you. You give energy to your past hurt by thinking about it again and again. If you ignore it, the thoughts of past hurt become weaker and weaker and finally disappear. You will be free from all past hurt. You will be free from the grudges, resentments, and negative emotions toward others and yourself. You will start your life anew. It's a second chance. In fact, every moment in your life is a second chance if you choose to let go of past hurt and live in the present moment.

> If you decide not to think about it, the hurt from the past loses its grip on you.

Do Not Intentionally Hurt Anyone

It is important that you do not hurt anyone's feelings intentionally. If you do so by mistake sincerely apologize. If anyone hurts you, forgive them so that you don't accumulate negative feelings within. Try not to cling on to the negative feelings toward anyone, because in the final analysis, those feelings cause more damage to you than to the other person. As Mark Twain said, "Anger is an acid that does more harm to the vessel in which it is stored than to anything on which it is poured." *If you want to keep your insides undamaged, remove all negative feelings about anyone and everyone from your heart!*

The Future: A Figment of Your Imagination

Your Inquiry into the Future Can Be Endless — Don't Fall into that Trap

When you think about the future, many questions arise. Will I ever be able to make enough money to live happily? Will I be able to afford good schools for my kids? How can I pay off my mortgage? What will everyone think about me in the meeting tomorrow? How do I convince my boss about the bonus? Will my marital relationship ever return to normal? How do I take care of my parents' health? What should I wear to the party? Will I ever fulfill my destiny? Our wandering minds can generate an infinite number of questions about the future if we allow them to.

Your Thoughts About the Future Are Generated in the Present

Most of these questions are genuine concerns; it is okay to ask them. But if you just ruminate over them, you won't find solutions. You will create stress. Move on and find solutions instead of worrying. You do not know what your future is going to look like. You are never going to know exactly what's going to happen next in your life. Then why get fixated on the future? Realize that your thoughts about the future are being generated in the present. The future you're thinking about is not here yet, you are just thinking about it.

A Calm Mind Will Guide You to a Bright Future

You tend to imagine a more fearful future than it actually turns out to be. In fact, the future is just a figment of your imagination; your entire future is in your mind. It has not happened yet, and it will not happen exactly as you imagine, either. There will always be things that affect your future more than you can understand or predict. So, why worry about things that you can't control? *Plan, set goals, and work from a calm state of mind. Let your inner wisdom guide you to the right opportunities and you will prosper. That's it! There will be fewer problems and less stress in your life!*

Do Not Imagine a Fearful Future because It Might Never Happen

To illustrate this point, see the following real-life example.

It was a hot summer day in May. I was diligently preparing for a medical exam called USMLE Step-2 the next day. For years, I had dreamed of becoming a doctor; I came to the United States for higher education. This exam was going to decide my future as a doctor in the United States. If I did well on the exam, my dreams would come true. If I didn't, it meant an end to my career here in the States.

I had been studiously preparing for the exam for almost six months while I was working toward my master's degree in public health and trying to make just enough money to live in a small dorm room I shared with another person. So, finally, exam day was here. I went to take the exam, nervous about whether I would fare well. It was an eight-hour exam with less than an hour break. It required lots of preparation, concentration, my being in a good state of mind, and the ability to perform well under pressure. I finished the exam to my satisfaction (at least I thought so). Now, I had to wait for a month before I got the results.

So, I waited impatiently, and each day felt like an eternity. I couldn't wait any longer … it was already three and a half weeks. Just another few days and I would know the result. But I could not wait any more. Someone told me that there was a secret way to find out whether I had passed the exam. If I went online and tried to apply for the exam again, and if the system blocked me from reapplying, that meant either I passed the exam or my result was not yet available. But if the system allowed me to reapply, it meant I had failed.

At that moment, I was ready to do anything to get over my apprehension about the result. Eagerly and anxiously,

I walked toward my desk, sat in the chair, closed my eyes for a moment, took a deep breath, and opened my laptop. My fingers were trembling with fear, but somehow, I was able to type in the required information to reapply for the exam. I was not really expecting it to go through … as I clicked the submit button, I was shocked to see the message on the screen, "YOU ARE ELIGIBLE TO REAPPLY."

For a moment, my mind went completely blank. I could not understand how this could have happened. I was in denial. I just couldn't believe it. I got a strange feeling in the pit of my stomach when I read this bad news. Slowly, a feeling of despair and deep sorrow started within. "Does this mean the end of my career? Does this mean that my two years of struggle and thousands of dollars spent for my education were in vain? How do I share this bad news with my family? What will happen to me now? Is my career over?"

A storm of negative thoughts enveloped me, creating a sense of insecurity about my future. My roommate, sitting a few feet away on the couch, noticed something was wrong. He had always been a keen observer and a sensible friend.

"What's going on? You look upset," he asked. I was so glad he asked me. I badly wanted to share this news with someone with the hope that it would ease some of the pain that I was feeling. I quickly explained the situation to him. He looked at me for a moment, and after a brief pause, he remarked, "I have known you for almost a year. You are a hard worker and you have always given the best you could. I don't believe you failed. Why don't you just wait for the official exam result by mail? Maybe what you saw on the computer is not true. Who knows?"

Well, those few words of solace and support gave me hope that maybe I had passed. The unofficial way of checking the result online is laden with mistakes. At that point, I had no choice but to wait for the official result.

The next few days were miserable. I was in such despair that I stopped doing everything else. I was imagining a very fearful future. I was thinking about all the debt I had accrued over the past two years, and how I would have to find some way to pay it all back. I was really taken aback by the fact that I had lost two years of my life for nothing. I would have to start my career all over again in India while my friends and fellow students were successfully reaching their goals and realizing their dreams here in the United States. My future looked dismal—there was no way out of the situation.

Three days later, I went down to the mailroom to see if my official exam report had arrived, and there it was. I opened the envelope with a sense of impending doom. My hands were shaking. As I opened it, again I was stunned— only this time it was very good news. I not only passed the exam, but had scored in the 99th percentile, the highest possible score! Tears started flowing down my cheeks as I walked back to my room. I was still looking at the document through my teary eyes to make sure that what I saw was indeed true and not my imagination.

After reading it up and down, left to right, and right to left, I was finally convinced that I indeed had passed the exam with the best possible score. I jumped up in joy, ran to the phone, and called first my roommate who had played a major role in the past few days in keeping my hopes up and calming me down. We celebrated that magical moment with so much joy that even today I remember those precious moments.

Now, as I was celebrating, I was also thinking, How foolish was it of me to imagine such a frightful future? I suffered all these days for nothing. It looked so real to me that I was in so much pain, yet it was just a figment of my imagination. It was all in my thoughts. If I chose wisely not to focus on these thoughts over the next few days, I would have avoided the anguish. Even if such a bad situation really arises, there is no point in worrying about it. Worrying never helps.

> There are always solutions for the problems we face in life. You may not be able conceive them right now but there are always solutions.

There are always solutions for the problems we face in life. You may not be able conceive them right now but there are always solutions. That day, I resolved to not fear the future no matter how dire my situation looked. Whatever happens will happen. When the time comes, I will have to face my future anyway, and I will. But, as of now, I am still in the present, not in the future. So just enjoy every moment you have today!

DR. CALM'S PRESCRIPTION

1 The past is nothing but a memory. Whether it happened a
✓ minute ago or a year ago, it is no more. However, you can
learn from your past.

2 Do not ruminate on your mistakes. The more you dig into
✓ the grave of your past, the worse you feel. Instead, remember
what is good, forget what is bad, learn from the experience,
and move on.

3 Give yourself and others a second chance. Mistakes do
✓ happen. If you hold on to past hurt, the one who suffers the
most is you!

4 Your future is not here yet. Realize that the future you think
✓ about exists just in your mind.

5 There are always things that will affect your future more
✓ than you can understand or predict. So, why worry about
what you can't control?

6 You can think, plan, and act to build a bright future. But
✓ you have to do that in the present moment.

7 Whatever you focus on, your mind makes it happen.
✓ So doesn't it make sense to focus on and project a more
optimistic future? Most people don't do that. They project
gloom and doom into their future, and thus create it.

CHAPTER 25

Sleep—The Secret Boon to Humanity

If not for sleep, humankind would not survive!

The Importance of Sleep

Volumes have been written about sleep and its importance in human life. In a few simple words, my message is: *Please do not ignore your sleep. Nothing in this world replenishes your energies like a peaceful, good night's sleep.* Most of us need around six to eight hours of sleep. You can live weeks without eating, but you can't function properly without sleeping even for a couple of days.

When sleep deprived, you feel irritable and even the most

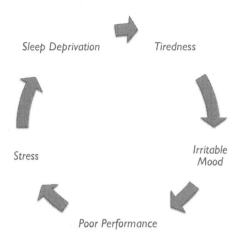

Figure 25.1. The Sleep Deprivation Cycle

melodious music can become a cacophony. Poor sleep makes your mind tired and error prone; you get into accidents and pose a danger to yourself and others. Your attention span and memory are affected, and you forget things easily. The list of bad effects due to sleep deprivation is endless (see Figures 25.1 and 25.2).

Good sleep is a must for a restful mind. A rested mind is a nest of calmness and clarity. So, each night, rest well. Don't you recharge your mobile phone every night so that you can use it the next day? Isn't that common sense? The same logic applies to recharging your body's battery. Make it a habit of having a deeply restful sleep to recharge and rejuvenate your mind-body battery. This will help improve your efficiency during the day. If you don't, you will always feel irritable. Why abuse your mind and body by depriving them of sleep and still relentlessly pushing them to work? Can you do the same thing to your phone? The phone will not function properly. In the same way, when you don't sleep well, your mind and body will stop working properly, too.

Some people lie in bed for six to eight hours or more but that doesn't mean that they have slept well. If you wake up periodically or have nightmares, you will have a poor night's sleep. To go

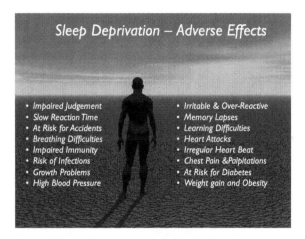

Figure 24.2. The Effects of Sleep Deprivation

back to the phone analogy, it's like removing your mobile phone from the charging outlet every few minutes throughout the night. Obviously, it won't be properly charged overnight. The next day when you go to work, it will work for a time and then shut off. Your body and mind will do the same thing if they don't have the sleep they need.

The Ten Commandments of Good Sleep Hygiene

1. Go to bed at the same time every night. Avoid interrupting that schedule as much as possible.

2. In the evening, avoid drinking caffeinated beverages (coffee, soda, etc.), high-energy drinks, excessive amounts of tea, or consuming any other substances that could over-stimulate your brain and interfere with your ability to fall asleep.

3. Do not bring the problems of the day into night. Do not lie in the bed thinking about them. A restless mind makes it difficult to fall asleep and maintain your sleep.

4. If you do have any problems you need to solve or think

about, do it well before you hit the bed. Make your bed a sacred place where you only use it for sleeping.

5. Empty your mind prior to going to sleep. Many things happen during the day that could affect your mind and fill you with restless thoughts. By purposefully setting aside a few minutes at the end of the day to totally relax and empty your mind, you can resolve that restlessness and sleep peacefully. The relaxation exercises discussed in this book can help with that.

6. Avoid watching TV at least for an hour prior to bedtime. Watching TV or any other visually stimulating events prior to sleep leaves an impression on your mind for a few hours, making it difficult to fall asleep and often resulting in disturbed sleep.

7. Avoid being drawn into the never-ending sensationalism of the news channels. Avoid arguments with friends, family, and neighbors, no matter how much you disagree over a topic. You can agree to disagree and be respectful to each other.

8. Excessive tiredness and stress can also make it difficult for you to sleep. So, keep stress at bay.

9. Avoid dependency on sleep medications. They may help you sleep well for a short time, but in the long term they can be detrimental to your health and sleep. Extended use of these medications can alter your brain hormones and make it difficult to fall asleep without using those particular medications every time.

10. Being at peace with yourself helps a lot. When your mind is peaceful, your sleep will be peaceful, too!

DR. CALM'S PRESCRIPTION

1 Sleep deprivation is not only detrimental to your mental health but also to your physical health.

2 A disturbed night's sleep shuts off your mind during the day. So, make every effort to have a deeply restful sleep every night. Make a firm commitment to that today.

3 A marker of good sleep is that you feel peaceful and rested after waking up. This good state of mind is essential to get you going with energy and enthusiasm all day!

4 Do not ignore your sleep at any cost! Sleep is the greatest healer. It recharges your body and mind every night. Without sleep, your body perishes faster than without food and water.

5 Respect your sleep time and sleep well. Sleep deprivation leads to irritability, mistakes, poor memory, reduced immunity, and related health consequences.

6 Understanding the Three Principles and practicing the relaxation exercises and the calming technique discussed in this book will help you sleep better at night.

7 When you have trouble falling asleep, try one of the relaxation exercises while lying in bed and you will relax, de-stress, and fall asleep soon.

Mastering the Big Three of Your Life: Time, Money, and Relationships

Part VII Objectives

- Accomplish more in less time: a new paradigm for time management
- Discover why money alone will not make you happy
- Learn the five keys to successful relationships

CHAPTER 26

Surviving the Time Crunch and Creating More Time for Yourself

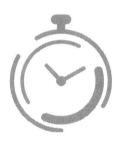

The only true measure of time is peace of mind. If you have peace of mind, all the time in the world matters. If not, every minute feels like hell.

Time Is Just an Idea in Your Mind

When we talk about absolutes, time is a misnomer. When we talk about relatives, time is a tool. Time is just an idea in your mind. If you are not thinking about time, time does not exist. How often in your life have you had the experience of having

Frozen Time   Broken Time

Frozen Time	Broken Time
☐ You are engrossed in the activity	☐ You feel bored and stuck
☐ You are totally enjoying the moment	☐ You are not enjoying the moment
☐ You lose track of time you spent	☐ You keep looking at the watch
☐ Time feels surreal	☐ Time looks real

Figure 26.1. Frozen Time vs. Broken Time

such a good time with your family or friends that time just flew by? You might have spent the entire day with them, yet it felt like just an hour. You did not look at your watch even once the whole day because you were thoroughly enjoying yourself, lost in time!

The Clock Is Merely a Tool. Don't Let It Dictate Your Life

Did you ever wait for a bus or train or got stuck in traffic and each minute felt like an eternity? You were so focused on the time that with each passing minute, you felt increasingly irritated. In your restless mind, time became a stress catalyst, rapidly creating the end product—frustration! But if you decide not to keep glancing at your watch, not to think about every passing minute, then you won't be frustrated. If you don't pay attention to it, then time won't bother you. But for one reason or another, too many people are stuck in this *time crunch* and make their lives miserable.

I am not saying time has no value. It has many practical uses, and that's all it is. *Time is just a tool, an idea, a medium of exchange all human beings use so that we can agree to a measurable unit of relative reality that holds us accountable to each other's schedules.* Yet, there are instances where we need to completely ignore time, as we discuss in the following sections.

Frozen Time vs. Broken Time (see Figure 26.1)

You are meeting a handsome teacher named Mark. You are supposed to meet him at a romantic and beautiful place of your liking. You go there with so much passion and enthusiasm and are just so excited to be meeting this person you fantasized about so much, and you are really hoping that this date will be successful.

Mark finally arrives. You warmly greet and hug each other. After a few moments of excited exchanges, you slowly walk together toward the table that was reserved for your first romantic dinner. As you sit down in the chair, you are very excited. You feel like all the time in the universe is frozen! You are so much enjoying each moment that time does not exist in your mind. You want this time to last forever.

As you lift your gaze and silently look at Mark, you are taken aback to find that a sense of excitement is missing in his face. He has been looking at his watch every minute, as if he is bored and impatient. It seems every minute that is passing by is taking your date away. You are now uncertain what's going on. "Why did this happen? What went wrong?"

A flood of restless thoughts pierce through the veil of joy you were floating in. Your frozen time now is broken. You are brought back from your world of eternal time to the world of relative time. You are no longer enjoying what was supposed to be a wonderful evening. Disheartened and deflated, you feel like ending the date and moving on.

After a long and boring dinner, which felt like an eternity, you finally set yourself free from that person, hastily walk toward your car, turn on your favorite music, and drive away from that place as fast as possible, hoping the feelings of disappointment and disheartenment will drift away!

Your Thoughts about Time Are More Important than Time Itself

Do you see how time is so surreal? One moment you feel like time is frozen, and the next you feel like time is an eternity. Time is a relative reality created by your mind. It's all in your mind. It's all in your thoughts. It's all in how you see and experience things. So, don't make time overly important. Know that it is a tool and use it that way. Once you are done using that tool, store it away. Live in the "now"! Enjoy the present moment. Know that your thoughts and perspective toward time is more important than time itself.

Time, Calmness, and Efficiency

The following real-life example illustrates the benefit that calmness has on efficiency.

Once, I was conducting a seminar, and at the end of it the vice president of human resources of the organization asked me, "How do we deal with stress related to time? It seems most of my stress comes from not having enough time in my day to get everything done."

I said reassuringly, "I can understand why you feel that way. You are not alone. Feeling short of time is a haunting problem for millions of people around the world. Our modern world is so fast paced that it seems twenty-four hours is not enough to complete our tasks every day."

"How do we solve this problem?" she asked, hurriedly looking at her watch, feeling stressed that she was getting late for work.

Sensing that she was in a rush, I quickly explained, "More than ever, we all are in a time crunch. 'Efficiency' is the new

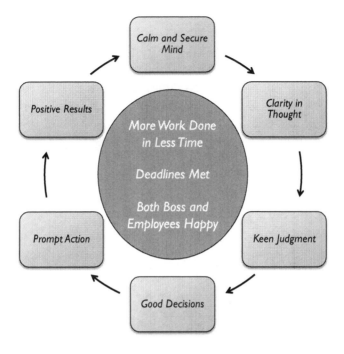

Figure 26.2. A Calm Mind Is Efficient

name of the game. We are conditioned by our demanding environment to achieve more in less time. But we are burning our candles on both ends, putting our physical health and mental peace at risk. The odds at stake are not worth it. This nonstop running around is often counterproductive, leading to stress, tiredness, and inefficiency."

I continued, "But there is a solution and it starts with asking ourselves, what is the reason for this time crunch? What has led us here? Is it our insatiable desire to achieve more in less time, or is it our restless minds that cannot work efficiently enough to finish the tasks scheduled in our day? What do you think?" I asked her.

After a moment, she thoughtfully answered, "I believe both play an important role. Currently, we are in a world where we all are being asked to do more in less time. Our workplaces have become dynamites of stress. The political dramas in our organizations, the tight financial bottom lines, the economic downturn, the failing social system, and declining moral and ethical values in society are all creating external pressures on us as individuals. We are stuck in a rat race, trying to run faster only to realize that seemingly there is no end to this game.

"Then how do you maintain your sanity while performing under pressure? How do you accomplish more in less time? How do you cut short the waste of resources?" There was a sense of urgency to her questions.

A Calm Mind Is Efficient (see Figure 26.2)

"The answer lies in having a calm mind," I remarked. "If you are calm, you can accomplish more in less time. When you are calm, your mind grasps things easily, comprehends them well, makes right decisions faster, which finally leads to good results. This is obvious to me both at work and home. On the days when I am calm and relaxed, I accomplish much more than when I am stressed. On the days when I am tired, stressed, and irritable, I spend long hours and accomplish less than I usually do."

Meanwhile, another member of the audience had joined us. He asked, "What should I do if I have a lot of work piled up and my boss is unhappy about it? How can I remain calm in that situation?"

I looked at this earnest gentleman in his thirties for a moment and said, "Regardless of the situation, there is no point in getting worried or restless. Only by being calm will you be able to finish your work on time. Imagine it takes two hours to perform a task in your office. If you are restless, it takes you three hours to finish the task and it is likely that you will make more mistakes. But if you are calm, you will be able to finish the same work in one hour's time with fewer mistakes. That saves you time and you prevent the overflow of work from one day to another. Your boss will no longer scold you because you are working efficiently and effectively. Over time, your boss will understand that you are calm, efficient, and effective, and on the rare occasion that you fall behind in your work, your boss is more likely to understand your situation. But if you are nervous and stressed all the time, keep missing your deadlines, and are inefficient, your boss might think you are a long-term slacker."

"That makes sense. Can you give an example of how a stressed mind is inefficient?" he asked.

Stress Breeds Inefficiency (see Figure 26.3)

"Sure," I replied. "Last year, I was involved in an important project that had a strict deadline. I was also working full-time as a physician. For almost two months, I was working nonstop both as a physician as well as the project leader. As a part of the project, I had to travel to San Diego, California, finish the project, and come back to

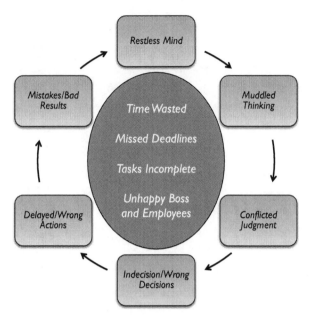

Figure 26.3. A Restless Mind Is Inefficient

Hartford, Connecticut, and resume my role as a physician at the hospital. I finished the project and came back the night before to Connecticut. I was very tired because I had been working nonstop for almost two months with very little time to relax. My mind was constantly working day and night to accomplish the goals I had set for myself to achieve. On top of it all, because of all the travel and with numerous flight delays with every trip, my sleep patterns became very erratic.

"I went to work Monday morning, and I was assigned to see the average number of patients I always see at the hospital, but as I worked through the day, I could feel that my energy levels were low. I ate well, I kept myself well hydrated, I went to work with the right attitude and enthusiasm, but I couldn't perform as well as I usually do. For every task I attempted, it took almost double the normal amount of time to accomplish. I had to take a break every hour to refuel my energy and refresh my mind. My mind could not concentrate at a peak level for more than an hour.

"I am usually very efficient at work and finish all my tasks much earlier than the allotted time. But this time, I noticed I was going home much later than normal. I asked my team to schedule less work for the next few days, and with their help, I finally finished that workweek. I decided at the end of the week to take off five days. My request was granted. I do not remember the last time that I had to make such a request. Those five days, I just relaxed completely. I did not work on anything else during that time. I practiced the P-E-T System, I slept more, read my favorite novel, went hiking, spent time in nature. And guess what happened?! Within three days, I was back to normal. I was rejuvenated. I de-stressed my mind and body. My mind became clear and composed. When I went back to work, I was at full capacity and efficient again."

Preventing Time Crunch

As they had this new insight about the relationship between time and a calm mind, both exclaimed at the same time with a sense of excitement and realization, "So, if I learn to be calm and relaxed, I can be efficient and prevent this time crunch?"

"Absolutely, yes," I said. The human resources executive

who had been concerned about time crunch earlier was no longer looking at her watch. She was interested in learning more and remarked, "Is calmness a habit? If we practice being calm most of the time, will it come to our rescue when we face challenges in life or when we are in a time crunch?"

The Habit of Calmness Will Come to Your Rescue

"Yes! Calmness will come to your rescue if you make it a habit!" I was excited that she had stepped out of the time crunch mode into the time freeze mode. I continued, "Recently, I was in that kind of situation. It was Sunday afternoon. There was a mild chill in the air; the skies were dark and cloudy, as if it were about to rain heavily. With the drought situation in California, rain was a much-welcome sign for all Californians. I was flying from Los Angeles to Boston after attending a medical conference. I was supposed to fly out from Los Angeles, California, to Hartford, Connecticut, that afternoon and reach home by Sunday night so that I could rest before I went back to work the next morning.

Not to my surprise, my flight was delayed. How many times in the past few years have I sat at the airport, watching the clock ticking because of delayed flights? If I added up all that time, it would easily equal my three-week annual vacation time. Nevertheless, I had to get on the earliest, next available flight so that I could reach home as soon as possible and be at work the next morning. After much difficulty, I was able to secure a flight that night around 10 p.m., which arrived in Boston the next day around 6 a.m. I could not get a flight to Hartford directly that night. That meant, after an overnight flight of six hours, I had to drive another two hours in morning traffic to reach Hartford.

I tried to sleep for a few hours on the flight, but the incessant announcements and uncomfortable seats meant a sleepless night. Tired and only half-awake, I finally reached Boston the next morning around 6:00 a.m. By the time I collected my luggage, rented a car, and left the airport, it was already 7:20 a.m. Time was ticking fast. In the rush-hour traffic on that Monday morning, somehow, I managed to keep my tired eyes open for the next two hours while driving home. I quickly took a shower, hastily gulped down a cup of orange juice, and swiftly pulled out of my garage to drive another forty minutes to finally reach my office around 10 a.m., which was very late. You can imagine my situation; I was extremely tired from a long flight, sleepless night, and a tiring, rush-hour drive. I thought when I got to work my problems would end there and I could somehow quickly finish my day. But fate had different plans. We unexpectedly had a workplace crisis that morning, which meant almost double the work than on a typical day at the hospital.

Peak Performance under Pressure

I thought, "I am dead. How can I perform under so much pressure, especially when I am sleepless and tired? I cannot believe my bad luck!" But as I started my workday and determined to do the best I could, I was pleasantly surprised to see that my mind was calm and clear, performing well even under extreme pressure. I managed to finish my work on time, went home that evening, and then crashed on the bed. I didn't wake up until the next morning after fourteen hours of deep sleep, catching up on the lost sleep from the night before.

The next day, when I woke up, it all felt like a dream. I was perplexed; how had I been able to remain unruffled and perform under tremendous pressure after an extremely tiring night on a coast-to-coast flight with minimal sleep and fatigue from driving? The only answer that I could think of was the power of the habit of calmness. The strong habit of calmness that I had developed over the years came to my rescue when I was pushed to my limits.

Chronic Fatigue Affects You

While these examples are somewhat similar (flying coast-to-coast from California back east, late flights, little sleep, going to work the next day), there are important differences. In this second situation, it is important to note that I was tired for only a short period (one day), unlike in the previous example, where I was tired for a long period of time (weeks to months). In the second situation, I did not accumulate a stress load over weeks and months as in the first example. That meant I was in a good state of mind over the past several months, so when a crisis erupted, my mind was prepared and relaxed enough to deal with it. But in the first example, because my mind was chronically tired and stressed, with many days of inadequate sleep, I could not even manage my routine tasks at an average efficiency.

The lesson to take away from these examples is, if you learn how to remain calm and stress-free most of the time, even under pressure, you will still be able to perform efficiently and effectively. But when you are chronically stressed, even a minor challenge can throw you off balance and make you inefficient. A mind strongly established in the habit of being calm can overcome the limitations of time and space!

> A mind strongly established in the habit of being calm can overcome the limitations of time and space!

Take a Break! And Don't Take Stress on Vacation with You

Stress has its own secret ways to enter your life. Sometimes, it happens because of your own accord, and sometimes it happens without your notice. Regardless, if you are self-aware and in touch with your feelings, you will recognize when you are getting stressed and tired. At that time, you can choose to relax and refresh. If you have to take a break, take a break. Don't let your pride override you. Don't let your ego prevent you from taking a well-deserved break. If you continue to drudge on, it will result in unnecessary mistakes. Be good to yourself.

Irrespective of how knowledgeable and skilled you are in your profession; a time will come in your life when you will feel tired and stressed. It's alright to feel that way. Acknowledge that fact. Know that you are not above nature and the natural limitations of your body. Do what is necessary to rejuvenate yourself. Do it without hesitation!

It is also important for you to know how to de-stress and relax when you go on vacation. It might sound strange, but many people go on vacation and come back even more stressed. They carry their work-stress along with them on vacation; get into an argument with their friend or family member; immerse themselves in too much drinking, smoking, or drugs; squander all their money stress shopping; and finally return from vacation feeling worse than ever. Deep inside, they feel miserable and guilty for using up their vacation time for nothing!

If you follow the P-E-T System, you will avoid this scenario. You will know how to remain calm, relaxed, and refreshed, whether on vacation or not!

DR. CALM'S PRESCRIPTION

1   ✓   In absolute terms, the concept of time is a misnomer. It is just an idea. In relative terms, time is a practical tool that can be used to carry out daily activities.

2   ✓   Preoccupation with time can kill your performance. Focusing too much on time can be counterproductive. Don't keep watching the clock and stress yourself!

3   ✓   It is not how much time you have but how you use your time that is more important.

4   ✓   A wandering mind squanders time. A focused mind can work wonders by efficiently using even the little time that's available. Poor time management is often the result of poor mind management.

5   ✓   Successful people do not wait until they have a lot of available time to accomplish their tasks. They make use of small "time gaps" in their calendar to drive toward success.

6   ✓   A restless mind is inefficient and lacks the necessary focus to finish the tasks at hand. To a restless mind, all the time in the world is not enough.

7   ✓   When you are calm, your thoughts will be organized, highly purposeful, and effective—thus accomplishing all tasks at hand efficiently. The little time you spend practicing calmness will save you a lot of time during the day.

CHAPTER 27

Less Stress, More Money: The Smart Way to Do It

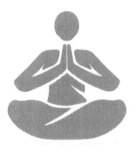

In the final analysis, wisdom is a treasure against time and will yield more wealth, health, and happiness than your dependence on money alone.

Is Money Bearing Your Burden, Or A Burden to You

Q. Money plays a huge role in our society and, thus, in our lives. Everything is linked to money. How is a lack or excess of money associated with stress?

A. Money by itself does not cause stress. Poverty is not necessarily a lack of money.

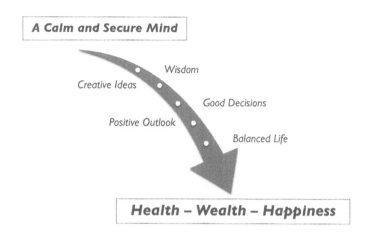

Figure 27.1. The Pathway to Health, Wealth, and Happiness

Poverty is mental scarcity and a lack of resourcefulness, and that is what causes financial stress. The poor mental world you live in causes stress. I personally know people who were born in poverty but used their talents to become financially well off. Depending on your environmental conditions, you may have to live in poverty for a little while, but you don't have to live there forever.

In today's world, everything is motivated by money. While money is needed to carry on life activities, money itself does not necessarily make you happy. People are so focused on money that they stake their peace of mind on the pursuit of wealth. They put their relationships at risk while chasing money. They don't hesitate to hurt others for the sake of material possessions. They lie and commit crimes for a few dollars. Yet, most people do not realize that *there is not always a cause-and-effect relationship between money and happiness*. Money and happiness are not always directly proportional to each other. Sometimes, they could be inversely proportional. Whereas too little money is not good, neither is too much money. As you focus purely on money and material accumulation, you forget about other important aspects of life. Soon, your life is out of balance and stress creeps in.

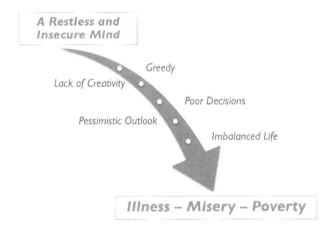

Figure 27.2. The Unwanted Pathway to Illness, Misery, and Poverty

Prioritize Peace of Mind

At best, it's reasonable to allot a certain amount of time and energy to the process of making money to secure your needs, but then spend the rest of the time building an inner fortress of peace, improving your relationships, spending time with your family, and doing things that bring true joy into your life. Keep peace of mind as your top priority in the hierarchy of values in your life. Do not lose sight of that priority for the sake of money or anything else. *Without peace of mind, you are poor even if you have a million dollars in your bank account.* Maintain a "peace-of-mind bank account" so that you can draw strength from it whenever you are in trouble. Strive for peace of mind first. If you have peace of mind, then having a million dollars will make all the sense in this world. But without peace of mind, a million dollars will not make you truly happy. It might give you transient pleasures, but not true happiness.

Q. Can you provide a real-life example of money and its effect on stress?

A. I will give you two examples.

Resourcefulness and a Positive Attitude Brings You More Success than Money

After I came to the United States, initially and for almost two years, I struggled to make money. I lived in a dorm with a friend (a single room, one bathroom, and a kitchen). I earned barely $900 per month, but I was extremely happy. I had a wonderful time and probably some of the best times in my life in those two years— great friends, great classmates, and great professors in college. Every now and then, I'd have a problem, but it was only transient. There were many expenses but somehow, I always met them. As I look back and evaluate that phase of my life, I realize it was my resourcefulness and positive attitude that helped me succeed and be happy during those times of financial hardship. Some of my classmates had better financial support but did not fare well and had to struggle a lot in their careers. The external circumstances were similar for all of us. Yet the internal environments of our minds were different and became the key factor determining our success or failure, happiness or distress, peace or restlessness.

Greed for Excess Money Causes Stress

Let me give you an example where my greed for excess money caused me stress.

After I became a successful practicing physician, I became well-off financially and was able to clear all my debts and my family's debts, too. I bought a house, and I gave money to various charitable organizations to help feed and educate the poor. But when I decided to make more money to buy a property, I started working extra shifts. Initially, I was happy. Money was flowing into my account, and I was soon gathering the necessary amount I needed to buy the property. But my schedule became so hectic I was working almost nonstop. Soon, my hectic work schedule started to affect my relationship with my wife. For a while, we spent very little quality time together.

It's very strange how subtly these things happen almost without your notice. You think everything will be okay but it won't be. Maybe we don't notice the minor changes in relationships until they become major problems. I was caught in the thick of it, focusing primarily on money making. I was out of balance. Also, this single-minded pursuit of money started to affect many of my other activities—my exercise routine and the time I would generally spend relaxing and meditating, and so on.

> Maybe we don't notice the minor changes in relationships until they become major problems.

Initially, when I observed that things were not going well in my life, I was not that concerned. I thought they would just get better on their own eventually. I was still meeting my other goal of making excess money to buy the property. But the longer I ignored the problem, the worse it got. I was feeling palpitations, nausea, and a sense of unease deep inside. Every day, I woke up with a heavy feeling of doom and gloom. My relationship with my wife became very strained to the point of breaking. I decided then to cut back on the number of hours I was spending at work.

If not for my understanding and application of the P-E-T System, I would not have salvaged the situation. It took extreme patience, resilience, love, kindness, and calmness to bring everything back to normal.

Do you see how I became very stressed because of my attachment to money? Having excess money does not automatically guard you from having stress. If you are greedy for money and material possessions, you will be blinded to other important areas of your life and you will damage them. *Greed makes you restless and shuts off your wisdom.* You start ignoring your conscience.

You make wrong choices and you lose balance in life. Stress starts finding its way back into your life.

Decide what your key priorities are in life and allot sufficient time to each of those areas. As long as you don't lose that balance, you can make as much money as you want to. *Money made in such a way brings harmony to your life. Money made at the expense of neglecting your relationships, health, and peace of mind brings disharmony to and wreaks havoc on your life.*

Q. So do you mean that having excess money or less money has no direct relationship to stress?

A. Yes. I know many people who have very little money who are happy. I know many people who have excessive amounts of money who are happy. I know people who have very little money and are miserable, and people with a lot of money who are in deep distress. *Money itself is not a stressor, whether in excess or small amounts. It is our attitude toward money and life that is the real determinant of our happiness.*

Why Are Rich People Unhappy?

Every day, as I walk through the hallways of the hospital where I work and see the janitors, transporters, and cleaning crews, they are always upbeat. I notice that they seem to be genuinely happy and completely enjoying themselves and their work. They are always singing and laughing and joking with their colleagues. On the other hand, I see a stark contrast between them and the nurses, doctors, and CEOs, who are very stressed. Maybe it is because of their sense of responsibility, excess work, or working in a highly litigious environment that causes their stress, but whatever the reason, the truth is they are more stressed than people who make less money. I consider it very sad that people who make a lot of money are unhappy. What is the purpose of all this money if it's not making you happy? I often remark to my friends and colleagues that it's not so much your external circumstances that determine your happiness but your own response to them. *If you learn how to control your internal world, the external world will not bother you so much.* We all live in our own mental worlds and experience them accordingly.

> If you learn how to control your internal world, the external world will not bother you so much.

Q. Do you think money can buy happiness?

A. My answer is yes and no. You need a certain amount of money to meet your basic needs, raise your kids, maintain your health, and other important needs in life. So yes, money can buy happiness to some extent. But after certain amounts, it might not increase your happiness by much. When people have excess money, they might spend it on the wrong things and might become slaves to bad habits like smoking, alcohol, and drugs.

Yet, at the same time, we all know that poverty can cause unhappiness, poor health, depression, a lack of educational opportunities, infant mortality, and a host of other problems. So, we should not live in poverty.

Live a Life of Simplicity, Modesty, and Resourcefulness

At best, I advocate the importance of living a life of simplicity, modesty, and resourcefulness. Strive to be financially comfortable, not necessarily extravagant. It is more important to adopt a mentality of abundance and resourcefulness. You should cauterize the habits of poverty and scarcity thinking. With willpower and the right attitude, you can earn enough to keep yourself happy. *It is important to know where to draw that line between using money to make yourself happy vs. misusing it to make yourself unhappy.* It is a very fine line, and it can only be recognized through wisdom borne out of practicing calmness. Life will test you, prod you, and lure you to make more and more. But you need to develop that sense of contentment and discernment to decide how much you

> Do not put your peace of mind and moral values at stake for money. If you do so, money will only bring you unhappiness in the end.

really need in your life. Once you decide that, you must make an honest and sincere effort to reach that goal through the right means. Do not put your peace of mind and moral values at stake for money. If you do so, money will only bring you unhappiness in the end. But if you make money through ethical and industrious means, it will bring you happiness. It will support your growth and success.

Q. How much money do I need to be happy?

A. Only your wisdom can answer this million-dollar question.

No amount of money can make you happy if you are miserable to begin with. Unless you change your attitude toward life, money might only accelerate your demise. There is no universal answer as to how much money each person needs. No amount of research can answer this question. In fact, the research keeps changing over time, providing a different answer at different intervals. The undeniable truth is that only the dictates of wisdom can answer that question. You need to make that decision based on your own unique needs, strengths, and limitations. You need to learn first how to intelligently evaluate your needs and priorities.

Your intelligence can be easily misguided if you are restless, and you might make wrong choices prodded by ego, pride, and comparing yourself with others. Therefore, *it is important that we all learn the art of finding calmness first in our lives so that the wisdom born of calmness will guide our intelligence to make the right financial decisions.* All our financial planning and investment efforts will give us good results if our- financial decisions are wise and provident. If our decisions are misguided, even wealthy people can become paupers very quickly. In today's world, we need to teach ourselves how to live by wisdom, not by fancy comparisons.

DR. CALM'S PRESCRIPTION

1 ✓ If money could solve all the problems in the world, then this world would be a very happy place. Unfortunately, it is not. There is so much suffering even in rich and developed nations.

2 ✓ Money is just a means to purchase something that you value. Money by itself has no value. It's a tool for exchange of one's appreciation for others' services.

3 ✓ An excess or a lack of money is not the sole determinant of your happiness. There are plenty of people who have little money but are very happy. Also, there are plenty of people who have a lot of money but are unhappy.

4 ✓ Money alone cannot create happiness, although it can enhance it. If you are a miserable person to begin with, all the money in the world may not make you happy but most likely it will lead you to more misery unless you work on changing your state of mind. Your happiness is manufactured within.

5 ✓ Greed leads to stress. Do not lose your peace of mind at any cost—even for a million dollars.

6 ✓ A life of simplicity and modesty combined with your resourcefulness will help you create abundant wealth to live happily. Avoid scarcity mentality; it is the harbinger of poverty.

7 ✓ Your inner wisdom is a treasure beyond measure. Your health is priceless. Protect both by living a stress-free life.

CHAPTER 28

Salvaging Stressed Relationships: The Five Essential Pillars

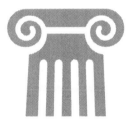

It's easy to love others when they love you. But it is hard to love people when they hate you. When you learn to love people who hate you, you will become the master of human relationships.

Why Do Relationships Become Complicated?

Many people are stressed because of bad relationships. Two people come together with the good intention of forming a union, whether it is wife and husband, boss and employee,

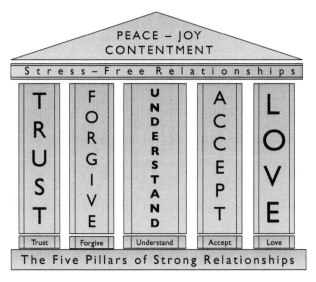

Figure 28.1. The Five Pillars of Strong Relationships

two friends, or any other relationship. But you soon find that the other person does not have what you are looking for, does not meet all your criteria for a good relationship, or they have different interests and viewpoints. Despite the initial good intentions, the relationship starts going downhill. Soon, you give up on it, thinking that if not this person, then another will fulfill your needs. But the fact is you will never find a "perfect" person who agrees with you about everything all the time. Remember, *perfect human relationships don't exist because we, as human beings, are imperfect.* Sooner or later, differences in opinions and problems arise. It is up to us how we resolve problems and reestablish harmony.

People often blame the relationships themselves and just say that relationships are complicated without realizing that it is their convoluted thinking that is making their relationships complicated. If your thinking is simple and straightforward, and you don't have ulterior motives, most of your relationships will become simple, enjoyable, and beautiful.

There are many attributes needed for building strong relationships. Below are the five essential pillars for building stress-free relationships (see Figure 28.1). I call them pillars because they provide the strong foundation on which beautiful relationships can be built. If any of these pillars, even just one of them, is weak, the relationship will start getting weaker. It finally may collapse unless corrective action is taken and the weak pillar strengthened again.

The First Pillar: Learn to be Understanding

Understanding is the anchor of strong relationships. *Try as you may, if there is no true understanding in a relationship, it will not last for long.* Who doesn't want a spouse who is understanding and supportive? Who does not want a friend who can see your viewpoint clearly? Who doesn't want a boss that is easy to get along with? We all do want such beautiful relationships that make our lives more enjoyable. Don't we? But, so many couples are getting divorced every day in this world because of that lack of understanding and rapport. Friends and colleagues get into conflict for the same reason. To gain such understanding, mental clarity is a prerequisite.

> Try as you may,
> if there is no true
> understanding in a
> relationship, it will
> not last for long.

Mental Clarity Is Essential for True Understanding

Restless thoughts make your mind clouded making it difficult to express yourself in a lucid manner. Ask yourself this question, "How can others see your viewpoint clearly if in your own mind you can't? Then how can you communicate your ideas clearly? You may think that you are expressing everything clearly, but others find it difficult to understand your viewpoint. When you practice the P-E-T System, mental clarity becomes second nature to you, and you will be able to express your thoughts with precision, making your ideas easily understood. This will equip you with the power to build rapport with others and enhance your personal and business relationships. But that only solves half the problem. The other half depends on how restless or calm the people you are communicating with. Unless they are clear headed, it does not matter how well you present your viewpoint. They still won't get it. A restless and clouded mind can't grasp things easily. Did you ever have the experience where you were trying as hard as you could to explain something to your spouse, friend, colleague, or client, but the person just did not get your point? Did you ever get into arguments and strain your relationships because of such instances? It is because one—or both of you—lack mental clarity.

Clear Your Mind before Important Discussions and Meetings

It is of paramount importance both in business and personal relationships to clear your mind of restless thoughts before you discuss important things. Practicing calmness for five minutes before each important meeting or discussion can significantly impact its quality and outcome. Also, before every meeting, take a few minutes to acknowledge that you all have different perspectives and limitations of understanding. That mutual acknowledgment will significantly impact the outcomes of your conversations whether at home or work.

The Second Pillar: Build Trust

There is no substitute for trust in relationships, and you develop them by walking your talk and talking your walk. In other words, have integrity. If you make a promise, keep it. If you can't, apologize and ask for forgiveness. Many relationships, both at home and work, are stifled because of a low trust environment resulting from backbiting, gossiping, having hidden agendas, and broken promises. There is only one way to solve the problems in our ailing relationships: build back trust. Be transparent, act with integrity, and avoid hypocrisy. Have good intentions at heart, keep calm, and do the best you can to serve whatever role you are given and ultimately things will work out. Remember that it takes time to build trust. So be patient and continue good work.

Trust Results from Being Open, Kind, and Honest

The best way to resolve our differences is to openly, honestly, and kindly communicate with each other. Some people express their differences openly and honestly but harshly. Harshness in tone and demeanor will only make the other person feel bad. It won't help. Also, harsh feelings within, even though not expressed aloud, can be felt by others. So, kindness is the key to success in relationships, along with honesty and openness. When we act like this, most people will understand us or at least try to understand us. If they do not, give them time. Give them space. Don't keep imposing your opinions on them if they do not want to listen to them. With time, most people come around and understand your sincerity in maintaining a good relationship.

Most important, when the other person is angry or upset and harsh with you, do not react to that. It won't help if you do. It only makes things worse. Refuse to participate in a discussion if the other person shouts or talks angrily. Maintain a strict silence (not an angry silence) in a nonreactive way or kindly excuse yourself and leave the scene. Again, kindness is the key here.

The Third Pillar: As Humans, We Are Imperfect—Learn to Forgive

No matter who the person is and what kind of situation you are in, always learn to forgive. Forgive yourself as well as the mistakes of others. As humans, we are imperfect. Every day, we make many errors of judgment, and our actions are not flawless. Sometimes, we are not even aware of the mistakes we commit. If not for the forgiveness of the people around us, we could not live a peaceful life.

Let Go of Resentment

Holding anger and resentment in your heart will only make things worse. Sooner or later, those negative feelings will come out in ugly forms such as divorce, loss of job, ill health or some other deadly consequence. So, let go of those negative feelings now! The person who holds negative feelings will be affected more severely than the person to whom those feelings are directed. Holding resentment within is like swallowing a deadly acid that scorches your insides. You must find an antidote for it, lest it's going to burn you down. The scorching fire of resentment can only be cooled down by the healing waters of forgiveness.

> The scorching fire of resentment can only be cooled down by the healing waters of forgiveness.

The Fourth Pillar: Acceptance Is Liberating

Forgiveness can't happen without acceptance. Practice acceptance. Acceptance is an essential step toward forgiving yourself and others. True acceptance happens only when you truly believe that everything happens for a reason. Know that a Divine Universal Plan exists. Like Master Oogway says in the movie *Kung Fu Panda*, "There are no accidents." There is always a bigger universal plan—even though we may not see it right now. When you come to terms with this truth, you will be able to let go of all negative feelings. And so, you will be able to heal yourself and find inner peace.

Sometimes, we love, trust, provide understanding, and forgive, but people might still not change and instead cause you even more trouble. You did all you could in your capacity to salvage the situation and improve the relationship, but you could not affect a good outcome. In those cases, accept them as they are. More importantly, come to a place of acceptance and peace in your heart. Let things be as they are. When they are ready to change, they will. You have to bide your time. As the serenity prayer observes:

> *God grant me the serenity*
> *To accept the things, I cannot change;*
> *The courage to change the things I can;*
> *And the wisdom to know the difference.*

The Fifth Pillar: Choose to Be Loving and Compassionate

When faced with a person who does something wrong or hurtful, ask yourself, "Why is this seemingly good person committing this wrong? He always has been good. Why is he being bad today?" If you take a moment to pause and ask this question, most of your anger toward that person will disappear. You can choose to be compassionate and understanding of that person's situation. But often that needs tremendous patience. Though most people are loving and compassionate by nature, many of them falter when it comes to patience. Because of that they appear to be lacking compassion. We all can learn to be more patient in the way we carry out our lives.

Patience Is a Virtue

The following real-life example illustrates the virtue of patience.

Once, I walked into a patient's room, and he was really sick. As I entered the room, he and his wife were very anxious. They started asking lots of questions and I answered them all, but they kept repeating the same questions. Even though I was composed and understanding initially, after some time, my patience started running out. But I did not express my impatience. I paused and thought to myself, "There must be something that's really bothering them. It seems they are looking for reassurance."

As I continued listening, they told me that their seven-year-old child was recently diagnosed with cancer and was getting chemotherapy. The man was feeling very frustrated, because instead of being at his child's bedside, he was stuck in the hospital. His wife had to divide her time between her husband and her child who were in two separate hospitals miles apart.

Once I was aware of their situation, my impatience vanished. I spent the next twenty to thirty minutes reassuring them and explaining things again in greater detail. Finally, when I saw that they were feeling better and more confident that things would improve, I was comfortable leaving the room. It's a deeply satisfying feeling for physicians when we truly make a difference in people's lives.

The important point here is that "patience is a virtue." Patience is an active emotion, and it takes more willpower than just not being upset or angry. If you have enough patience, you can turn all your enemies into your friends. But often we lack it. That's the reason people get into trouble. *Those who practice patience become invincible to the lashes of fate.*

Practical Application

The Mantra for Successful Relationships

Avoid assumptions, clarify when needed, and always try to understand. Without true understanding, love cannot flourish, and human relationships perish. True understanding comes from being curious about other people's perspectives without being judgmental. *When understanding is established between two hearts, even the most difficult conflicts dissolve instantly and upset feelings are replaced by feelings of love and kindness.*

Do Not Give Feedback when People Are in a Defensive Mode

Even after doing all these things with the best of intentions, some people will take your feedback or opinion in a negative way. This is because deep within themselves they are insecure. They thrive on people always telling them that they are good. When critical feedback is given or when their weaknesses are exposed, they feel vulnerable. They become defensive. They will do all that is possible to prove that they are right and will justify their behaviors and actions with a multitude of reasons. You can't win them over. You won't be able to convince them of the point you are trying to make. All your good intentions and good reasoning will fall on deaf ears.

The key in such scenarios is to give them understanding. Do not react in a way that provokes them or makes them feel more vulnerable. You have to understand that it is their insecurity that is making them behave this way. When you truly understand them and continue to be kind toward them, they will eventually get to know you better. They will feel that you are not a threat to them. They will start trusting you even though they may not trust others. Once that trust is built, you will have a better chance of positively influencing them.

Stay Away from Deceitful People

There are other kinds of people who seemingly look friendly and helpful, but given the slightest opportunity, will backstab or deceive you. (By *deceive*, I mean knowingly harm the people who trust them.) These are the most dangerous people you should be wary of. *It is not the openly straightforward and emotional people who you have to worry about, but the deceitful people you must be very cautious of.* Emotional people are usually straightforward, and you know what to expect from them and can prepare yourself to deal with them. But deceitful people are constantly plotting behind your back, and you never know what kind of plot they're brewing. At best, it is important to avoid these people. How do you identify them? They are dishonest, mistrustful, and do not hesitate to harm others for their own good. If you see such qualities in a person, stay away from him or her. If your job or situation requires you to be in their vicinity, keep contact to a minimum and businesslike without disclosing any important personal information. *You can be friendly, but you don't have to be friends.* Over time, if you see them change, then you might consider developing a personal relationship; if not, keep your distance.

How to Deal with Dishonest People

There are other kinds of relationships where you find people to be dishonest but not necessarily harmful or deceitful. They may be dishonest either because they haven't developed strong moral values since their childhood, or they are too insecure to be honest and open, or they might fear being judged, or for any other reason. You know that it is wrong to be dishonest, and if they are receptive, you can help them. You can lead them by example. You can give them a helping hand. They can benefit from your friendship. But you must make sure not to fall to their low standards and become like them. *Influencing and transforming other people is not an easy task. It takes great moral authority and unshakeable character.* If you have this in you, you will start impacting other people's lives positively, even if you don't know it.

No One Likes to Be an Emotional Wreck

There are other kinds of people who are well intentioned but are emotionally labile and become stressed easily. They often have emotional outbursts, say mean things, or act inappropriately. Be compassionate toward them. Try to see that they do not enjoy being emotional wrecks all the time. They suffer being that way. They are more miserable than the people they affect. Expressing compassion and truly caring for their well-being will help them tremendously. True understanding can literally change them completely. Be that person who provides true understanding and support for them if you are emotionally strong. It's a noble thing to do.

Everything Is Thought

In the end, realize that all your experiences are born out of your own thoughts. That realization will help you find your way back to mental well-being. No matter what people say, do, and think, realize that it is just *thought*. Everything originates from thought, whether people are doing things consciously or not. If you can hold onto that truth, you will remain emotionally unaffected regardless of what people say or do.

The following real-life example illustrates the above point.

> One day, my wife and I were sitting at home discussing nothing in particular. After a few minutes, our conversation led to a difference in opinion, and we got into a serious argument. We both held tight to our side of the argument and to what we held to be the truth. After a while, both of us were frustrated and angry. You could feel the tension in the room. I stopped arguing and sat quietly for a few minutes on the couch. Five minutes later, a deep insight stuck me so strongly that I started laughing. I realized that whatever argument we were having, it was all thought. All the content of the argument, perceptions, truth, and

everything in the situation arose out of our own thoughts. There was no other reality than what each of us thought about the situation. We created our own thoughts, our perceptions, our truths, and held tightly to them and then defended our thoughts, which led to the argument.

As soon as I realized this, all the negativity in my mind lost its momentum and dropped away. Almost instantly and effortlessly, a smile appeared on my face. My wife was silently observing the transition of my emotions from anger to withdrawal to deep introspection to confusion to the realization of truth and then to the smile on my countenance. In those five minutes, as I started laughing uncontrollably, a faint smile appeared on her face as well that soon grew wider and wider. She started laughing, too. She did not know what was happening in my mind, but my positive energy was contagious. After a few minutes of uncontrollable laughter, I explained my realization to her.

In every difficult experience, there lies an opportunity to learn something if you are ready to look within and if you are willing to calm down and honestly examine your thoughts and intentions. Please do not be discouraged when you face challenges, meet obstacles, or experience negative situations in life. Just take steps to calm down and you will find solutions. It can happen in any moment. Your mental well-being is always just an insight away.

> Your mental well-being is always just an insight away.

DR. CALM'S PRESCRIPTION

1. Understanding each other in a relationship is a prerequisite for lasting love. With misunderstanding, even the closest relationships perish. But with true understanding, even conflicted relationships heal and flourish.

2. Mental calmness and clarity are prerequisites for proper understanding. If your mind is restless and distracted, you won't be able to comprehend the real meaning behind people's words and their emotions.

3. Know that your thinking will directly influence your relationships. If your thinking is complex, your relationships are also going to be complex. If your thinking is simple, straightforward, and without guile, your relationships will also take on that form.

4. Treachery is the greatest sin in relationships. Never be deceitful to those who trust you.

5. Openness, kindness, honesty, and lack of prejudice wins you lasting friendships; a calculated, careful, materialistic approach toward people will only gain you short-term acquaintances.

6. Forgiveness is healing, acceptance is liberating, and compassion is uplifting. Embrace these great qualities and inspire others.

7. In the end, realize that every idea, concept, perspective, and judgment you have about any relationship is your own interpretation about it at that moment in that state of mind. Realize that all your life experiences are born out of your thoughts. Knowing this will help find your way back to mental well-being.

A Paradigm Shift for an Emerging Era of Calm

*"People don't care how much you know, but
they know how much you care."*

~THEODORE ROOSEVELT

Become a Peace Multiplier

The prize of regularly practicing the P-E-T System is peace of mind. A state of peace often attracts grace, which is closely followed by abundance in life. The fastest way to multiply that peace of mind and abundance is to share it with others. Share with people what you have. Direct them to find peace and joy in their lives. Be the peace multiplier. Be loving, kind, and compassionate. Do not try to show off what you have. Do not try to prove to others how much you know. Remember, in the end, beyond all the knowledge you have, it is love, kindness, and compassion that matter the most. After all, as Theodore Roosevelt remarked, *"People don't care how much you know, but they do know how much you care."*

Do Not Be a Constant Complainer

Most people complain about the things that are wrong with their environment and yet they do not make any positive contribution to make it better. They live in those same stressful surroundings every day and endure them all their lives. A conflicting and contentious environment drains your energy and requires tremendous willpower to remain calm and centered. Wouldn't it be helpful if your environment was conducive to peaceful living and the people around you were kindhearted, joyful, and optimistic instead of having an atmosphere full of conflicts? Not only do you want this, but everyone around you wants the same thing.

Be the Beacon of Light

Then instead of being one of those complainers, why don't you be the change agent and be the beacon of light? Do whatever you can in your capacity to make this world a better place to live for yourself and those around you. Even a little positive effort, if carried out with sincerity and regularity, can bring enormous positive change. Sometimes, the effect is immediate and at other times it's more insidious. You can start with simple, kind gestures to your fellow human beings, such as having a genuine smile on your countenance, being appreciative of others' good qualities, or sending good wishes to them. You may not be aware of it, but those simple, kind gestures have a lot of power.

You can't give solace to others if you yourself are constantly stressed in your own life. Your ability to shower peace, love, and joy on others is directly proportional to your ability to remain peaceful, joyful, and content within. Like a destitute person who can't donate money, if you are a destitute of peace and happiness, you can't help others to be peaceful and happy. People who lack peace of mind are often so consumed by their own thoughts that they have little time and energy to help others around them.

First, Find Peace for Yourself

So, the first step to becoming a peace multiplier is to find that peace of mind for yourself. When you have it, you will spread it around effortlessly. You will be like a rose flower spreading its fragrance all around without trying hard. Even though it doesn't do it on purpose, a rose can't stop spreading its fragrance. In the same way, if you are a peaceful soul, you can't help but ooze that peace, joy, and love, and the people around you will feel it. They will be uplifted and influenced by your calm and composed presence. You will enrich the lives of others along with enriching yours.

The New Beginning — The Stress-Free Revolution

In this process of becoming stress-free and finding peace of mind for yourself, you will develop enough strength that you can fulfill your duties, goals, and dreams. In your efforts to keep yourself stress-free, you become a part of a Stress-Free Revolution aimed at alleviating the suffering of people across the globe and elevating their emotional well-being.

To learn more about this stress-free movement and to be a part of it, email info@StressFreeRevolution.com.

ABOUT THE AUTHOR

Dr. Kiran Dintyala grew up in India and was inspired to enter medicine after his sister was diagnosed with cerebral palsy. Wanting to be able to help his sister and fulfill his lifelong dream, Dr. Dintyala attended medical school in India before entering West Virginia University to earn his master's degree. Like most people, Dr. Dintyala has had several periods of hardship in his life and career—from trying to finish graduate school to his early years as an intern at a demanding New York hospital. During the past fifteen years, he has dealt with many extremely stressful situations including deep financial troubles, unexpected death of loved ones, career crises, health and relationship struggles and much more. More than ten years ago, he stumbled upon powerful principles and techniques that helped him find *'Calm in the Midst of Chaos'* and turn around difficult situations and went on to have a successful career and a growing family.

An author, speaker, and stress management expert, Dr. Dintyala is the founder of Stress-Free Revolution. His mission is to alleviate the suffering and improve the emotional well-being of people across the world, and to raise the global happiness index.

Dr. Kiran Dintyala is a board-certified internal medicine physician practicing in San Diego, California. He holds a master's in public health (MPH) and an MD in internal medicine. He is also a Diplomate of the American Board of Integrative and Holistic Medicine.

In leisure he loves to watch movies, listen to music, and read books. He enjoys singing and spending time in the nature. Now that he has finished this book, he is looking forward to taking a vacation with his family and is planning to spend a lot more time near the beach.

BRING DR. CALM TO YOUR NEXT EVENT

If you would like to invite Dr. Calm for a speaking engagement at your organization, please telephone 858-869-0894 or send an email to Dr.Calm@StressFreeRevolution.com.

If you would like to set up a personal appointment with Dr. Calm, he is available at his Stress Management and Wellness Clinic in San Diego, California. He is also available for one-on-one consultations over the phone or Skype. For more information, please email info@StressFreeRevolution.com or telephone 858-869-0894.

About Speaking Presentations

Keynote

Exclusively designed and refined to create the most powerful impact in the least amount of time, Dr. Calm's signature keynote presentation takes the audience through a stunning set of illustrations and slides.

Combined with his calming presence, this 40-minute presentation invokes deep peace, joy, and meaningful insights that are life-changing.

Just sit back, relax, and watch the show. You are sure to be thrilled!

Seminars and Retreats: The Stress Mastery Program

Explore the P-E-T System for Stress-Free Living®. Transform your life forever with a calming and insightful interaction with Dr. Calm.

You will be able to discuss and understand a wide variety of topics from acute vs. chronic stress, internal vs. external sources of stress, and the true vs. false sources of stress in your life.

As you uncover these teachings, a natural and simple understanding dawns upon you that will guide you to the long- sought shores of happiness and success in life.

We will practice relaxation exercises and calming techniques together, and I will personally train you to master these techniques.

You will feel a sense of freedom from all worries, fear, and anxiety in your life. You will finally be able to learn to let go of any negative emotions harbored in your heart.

Ultimately, a natural peace, joy, and contentment will fill your being from within—your life will be completely trans- formed. Don't miss it!

For more information, please telephone 858-869-0894 or send an email to info@StressFreeRevolution.com.

Further Reading

- *The Missing Link*, by Sydney Banks
- *Where There is Light*, by Paramahansa Yogananda
- *Jonathan Livingston Seagull*, by Richard Bach
- *Synchronicity*, by Joseph Jaworski
- *The Seven Habits of Highly Effective People*, by Stephen Robert Covey
- *Notes to Myself*, by Hugh Prather
- *The New Earth*, by Eckhart Tolle
- *A Master Guide to Meditation*, by Roy Eugene Davis
- *Autobiography of a Yogi*, by Paramahansa Yogananda
- *Why Zebras Don't Get Ulcers*, by Dr. Robert Sopolsky

Made in the USA
San Bernardino, CA
10 January 2019